DIRECT MYOCARDIAL REVASCULARIZATION: HISTORY, METHODOLOGY, TECHNOLOGY

Developments in Cardiovascular Medicine

Previous volumes are still available

KLUWER ACADEMIC PUBLISHERS - DORDRECHT/BOSTON/LONDON

DIRECT MYOCARDIAL REVASCULARIZATION: HISTORY, METHODOLOGY, TECHNOLOGY

Edited by

Peter Whittaker, Ph.D.
George S. Abela, M.D.

KLUWER ACADEMIC PUBLISHERS
Boston/Dordrecht/London

Distributors for North, Central and South America:
Kluwer Academic Publishers
101 Philip Drive
Assinippi Park
Norwell, Massachusetts 02061 USA
Telephone (781) 871-6600
Fax (781) 871-6528
E-Mail <kluwer@wkap.com>

Distributors for all other countries:
Kluwer Academic Publishers Group
Distribution Centre
Post Office Box 322
3300 AH Dordrecht, THE NETHERLANDS
Telephone 31 78 6392 392
Fax 31 78 6546 474
E-Mail <orderdept@wkap.nl>
Electronic Services <http://www.wkap.nl>

Library of Congress Cataloging-in-Publication Data
A C.I.P. Catalogue record for this book is available
from the Library of Congress.

Direct myocardial revascularization : history, methodology, technology/edited
by Peter Whittaker, George S. Abela.
    P. Cm -- (Developments in cardiovascular medicine : 211)
Includes index.
ISBN 0-7923-8398-2) (alk. Paper)
    1. Transmyocardial laser revascularization. 2. Transmyocardial laser
revascularization. 3. Myocardial revascularization.
    I. Whittaker, Peter A., 1939-   . II. Abela, George S.
    III. Series.
        [DNLM: 1. Myocardial Revascularization--methods. 2. Myocardial
Revascularization--instrumentation. 3. Laser Surgery. WG 169 D598 1998]
RD598.35.T67D56 1998
617.4' 12--DC21 DNLM/DLC
for Library of Congress   98-47455
                                                              CIP

Contents

"With reference to the narrative of events, far from permitting myself to derive it from the first source that came to hand, I did not even trust my own impressions, but it rests partly on what I saw myself, partly on what others saw for me, the accuracy of the report being always tried by the most severe and detailed tests possible. My conclusions have cost me some labor from the want of coincidence between accounts of the same occurrences by different eye-witnesses, arising sometimes from imperfect memory, sometimes from undue partiality for one side or the other. The absence of romance in my history will, I fear, detract somewhat from its interest; but I shall be content if it is judged useful by those inquirers who desire an exact knowledge of the past as an aid to the interpretation of the future, which in the course of human things must resemble if it does not reflect it."

Thucydides. Peloponnesian War, Book 1.

PREFACE

The last five years have witnessed an increasing interest in the subject of transmyocardial laser revascularization (TMR) as illustrated by the number of abstracts presented at the meetings of the American Heart Association and the American College of Cardiology (Figure). The ideas and concepts associated with this particular method of myocardial revascularization have changed dramatically over even this short period of time. The original premise of "de-evolving" mammalian hearts to recreate a reptilian-like myocardial circulation by making multiple channels through the myocardium has been almost (but perhaps not quite) completely dismissed. Now, the most popular notion is that there is an angiogenic response to myocardial channel making. It is this development of new blood vessels that is thought to be responsible for the apparent improvements in symptoms and blood flow. Along the way, the idea that a channel could stay open and allow blood to flow directly from the ventricular chamber has found little support. Rather than directly explore all of these issues and merely duplicate previously published articles, our aim was to take a novel approach: that is, to step back from these arguments and provide perspective from the vantage point of distance. In the case of transmyocardial revascularization, distance comes both in terms of history and in terms of methodology and knowledge from other fields of research.

Historically, innovative methods of myocardial revascularization are by no means uncommon. The first two chapters deal with this historical perspective. There is undoubtedly something to be gained from knowing what advances and, even more importantly, what mistakes were made in the past. In this respect, it is interesting to note that approximately 15,000 patients were treated with the Vineberg procedure before it was abandoned in favor of coronary artery bypass graft surgery (chapter two). Thus, the historical context of transmyocardial

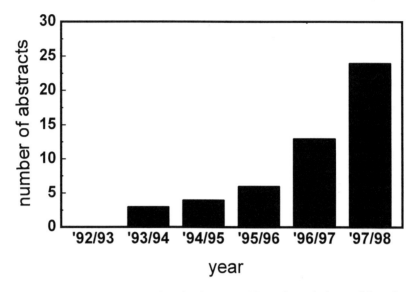

Figure 1. Abstracts presented at the American Heart Association and American College of Cardiology annual meetings in each "season" from 1992/1993 onward. The abstracts were indexed under the heading of "laser".

revascularization should be appreciated before we hail it as the "next big step forward". It is perhaps also prudent to note that the increase in the number of TMR abstracts illustrated in the figure was matched by a corresponding decrease in the number of abstracts on the subject of laser angioplasty. Does a similar fate await TMR?

Even amongst surgeons who are frequently more willing than most to try new devices and techniques, some of these innovative techniques were treated with considerable skepticism because the methods appeared to be based on questionable physiologic foundations. Professor Pifarré raised serious misgivings about the so-called myocardial acupuncture method (the original TMR procedure) when it was introduced in an attempt to revascularize hearts more than thirty years ago. Even though "high-tech" lasers have now replaced "low-tech" needles, Professor Pifarré has seen nothing to change his mind about the validity of such methods as he revisits his original paper in chapter three. Before TMR can be fully accepted as a legitimate revascularization method, the questions regarding mechanism must be answered.

The methodology required to evaluate TMR has, by necessity, been drawn from extremely diverse areas of both clinical and basic research. In this context, one of our surgical colleagues has often wondered what useful work ever came out of "academentia". Although it is true that many surgical advances have come through direct on-the-job experience, it would be unwise to dismiss basic experimental studies and their methodology completely. An understanding of the mechanism(s) by which TMR works may well come from animal studies; however, the methodology and design of such experiments, in addition to the end-points used to assess efficacy are perhaps not well known to investigators outside this area of experimental cardiology. Thus, chapter four describes the advantages and disadvantages of different models designed to evaluate methods of treating ischemia in both acute and chronic situations. Chapter five describes one approach that has been used to assess perfusion in such models; a vital step in evaluating TMR. Technological issues related to the use of different laser wavelengths for TMR and the prospects for making the channels from inside the heart are addressed in chapter six. Although the reasons behind the choice of the high-power carbon dioxide laser for the first clinical trial (described in chapter eight) are logical, there is a distinct possibility that there may be a more appropriate choice. That most studies have failed to demonstrate open channels when examined weeks or months after they were made may indicate that appropriate methods have yet to be employed. Chapter seven illustrates that open channels can in fact be found and suggests that the channel-making method may be crucial.

The clinical TMR studies are not reiterated in detail here for several reasons. First, they have been remarkably consistent and uncontroversial in their findings (primarily a rapid and marked reduction in angina) no matter where the study was performed or what type of laser was used. Nevertheless, we have included a historical perspective on the first clinical trial in chapter eight, in addition to details of some of the on-the-job lessons that the surgeons received. Secondly, the clinical data illustrating improved perfusion after treatment is at best equivocal, which is rather surprising for a treatment that was (is) intended to revascularize the myocardium. Chapter nine illustrates evidence of improved perfusion in a case report. Measurement of perfusion requires an appreciation of methodology, primarily from the field of nuclear imaging. Thus, chapter ten describes what can and cannot be expected from nuclear studies.

One of the current concepts in the field of TMR research is that the channel-making process stimulates angiogenesis. As attractive and compelling as this idea is, it does bring in yet another variable into the equation and an additional set of methods. Perspective from this area of research and its implications for TMR are discussed in chapter eleven.

In this preface, we have used the abbreviation TMR. However, some of the authors used different abbreviations; sometimes more than one in the same chapter. In editing the book, we made no attempt to standardize the usage. This variability illustrates the different perspectives and perhaps even biases involved. For example, TMLR is often used, but lasers are not be the only, and perhaps not even the best, device to use. In addition, it is no longer true to say that the procedure is always transmyocardial, and we have already commented on the issue of whether or not there is good evidence that "R" should be used. For these reasons, we finally opted for the title, "**Direct Myocardial Revascularization: history, methodology, technology**". We hope that the information provided here will provide the necessary perspective to stimulate investigators (both clinicians and basic scientists) to ask the appropriate questions in their own experiments and, in time, determine whether direct myocardial revascularziation has a place in the treatment of coronary artery disease.

1

EARLY METHODS OF MYOCARDIAL REVASCULARIZATION

Bernard L. Tucker

Good Samaritan Hospital, Los Angeles, CA

INTRODUCTION

Heberden, when he made the classic description of angina pectoris in 1772, was not concerned about the relationship between the anginal syndrome and coronary artery disease [1]. Over the next one hundred and fifty years, the understanding of the pathology, pathophysiology, and the clinical correlation slowly evolved. By the early 20th century, the clinical presentation and consequences of sudden coronary artery occlusion were recognized [2]. However, surgery of the heart was in its infancy. Rehn in 1896 had sutured a cardiac laceration, and ten years later Trendelenberg performed surgery for massive pulmonary embolus. The 1920's saw mitral valve surgery begun by Souttar and Cutler [3]. It was in this setting that the first procedures designed to treat patients with myocardial ischemia were developed.

INDIRECT PHYSIOLOGIC ALTERATIONS

The first operations were indirect methods to either influence the pain of myocardial ischemia by the interruption of sensory nerve pathways, or to decrease the cardiac workload by lowering the body's metabolic requirements.

The first surgical attempt to positively influence the pain of angina pectoris began early this century. Following a suggestion in 1899 by Francois-Franck [4], Jonnesco reported in 1920 an extensive operation performed four years earlier on a 38-year-old man to remove three cervical and the first dorsal sympathetic ganglia on the left side [5]. This sympathetic denervation had a sound physiologic/anatomic basis, namely the interruption of stimuli originating in the ischemic heart which are carried to the spinal cord. These impulses normally overflow and stimulate the somatic neurons of the thorax, neck and arms. This relatively extensive procedure interested many surgeons, but was unpopular because of its complexity.

In 1923, Coffey and Brown, of San Francisco, reported on a series of five patients, wherein either the superior cervical sympathetic ganglion alone, or the main branch from the ganglion to the heart was resected [6]. This operation was attended by a lot of interest because of its relative simplicity, and became a popular surgical approach to patients with angina.

Cutler, in 1927, in a comprehensive review article titled, "Summary of experiences up to date in the surgical treatment of angina pectoris," reviewed the various ablative procedures advocated by that time including the Jonnesco operation, procedures on the cervical ganglion only, the vagus nerve, and posterior rhizotomy [7]. Surgeons differed in their choice of a specific procedure and how best it should be performed and how extensive it should be. Since pain was the chief symptom, these procedures did not lend themselves to animal experimentation. Cutler cautioned on the difficulty of interpreting the results of the published reports, because the data in some instances were so meager. He conceded that in some operations, it could be difficult, even impossible, to verify the ablation of all the sensory pathways coming from the heart. The "psychic element" of angina pectoris also cast doubt on the interpretation of results. His review showed that 80% of the patients were improved. Some investigators even hoped that nerve ablation increased circulation to the heart by coronary vasodilation; however, eventually everyone believed the results were entirely due to elimination of afferent pain fibers. Despite often encouraging results, cervical and thoracic sympathectomy eventually gave way to procedures that promised to increase myocardial blood flow.

Thyroidectomy was the other indirect surgical method used to treat angina. Blumgart, in 1933, reported an experience with thyroid ablation to treat congestive heart failure or angina [8]. He referred to observations made, a century earlier, on the cardiac manifestations of exophthalmic goiter. This hypothesis was based on studies of the velocity of blood flow in health and in the thyrotoxic state, and the observation that thyrotoxic patients in congestive heart failure become compensated after subtotal thyroidectomy. The possibility occurred to Blumgart that euthyroid patients with congestive heart failure might improve if their metabolic rate were lowered. His report cited at least ten patients treated by thyroidectomy; two of the patients had angina pectoris by all available clinical criteria. These latter two patients with angina were symptomatically much improved following subtotal thyroidectomy. He attributed the benefits to a decreased amount of work performed by the heart, a decrease in its metabolism, and perhaps the decreased sensitivity of the heart to epinephrine. The operated patients were not incapacitated by the symptoms attendant to surgically induced hypothyroidism. He did, however, caution about possible injury to the recurrent laryngeal nerves, and the parathyroid glands. He cautioned about the widespread use of the technique, and advocated strict criteria that should be offered to a relatively small group of patients observed over a long period of time.

Thyroidectomy became popular [9,10] until the operation was supplanted by the availability of the antithyroid drugs, including radioactive iodine. The results using these medical thyroid suppressants were often inconsistent or equivocal. So, like sympathectomy, thyroidectomy was virtually abandoned when early results of the operative efforts to increase myocardial blood flow were judged promising.

As late as 1967, Braunwald et al advocated electrical stimulation of the carotid sinus nerve to control angina [11]. It was postulated that such stimulation abolishes angina by lowering the heart's energy requirements: heart rate, myocardial contractility and ventricular pressure. This modality of treatment had limited use and was quickly overshadowed by the tremendous amount of interest and success with coronary artery bypass surgery evolving at that time.

AUGMENTATION OF CORONARY CIRCULATION

Indirect Myocardial Revascularization

Disappointed with the results of the indirect methods to treat angina pectoris, and pressured by a desire to increase the blood supply to the heart, the decade of the thirties saw much activity, first in the laboratory, and then clinical applications. Simultaneously, investigators were working on the same or different time-consuming animal research. Results were often difficult to evaluate; trials in humans and animals often differed. Clinically, the outcomes could span the range between excellent and complete failure. So intense and widespread were these investigations, it is often difficult to assign credit to any particular investigator for having performed the first procedure of any kind, since many were pursuing the same course in different countries, and indeed even in different parts of the same country. One of the methods developed, the Vineberg procedure, is described in detail in one of the other chapters and so I will not discuss it here.

Claude Beck first tackled the problem of bringing a new blood supply to the heart; he continued this endeavor all his life. In 1932, Beck observed that in experimental pericarditis, the resulting adhesions between the pericardium and epicardium were vascular [12]. In 1934, while operating on a patient with chronic pericarditis, he observed bleeding from the cut ends of adhesions. His impressions were encouraged by a series of reports beginning with Langer [13], who, in 1880, outlined the Thebesian venous system of the heart and demonstrated communications between the coronary arteries and vessels of the parietal pericardium, mediastinum, diaphragm, and hila of the lung.

It was shown that obstruction of a coronary artery promoted the development of inter- and intracoronary collaterals, as well as collaterals from the systemic circulation through the mediastinum. Beck stated that these vessels made it possible for blood to get to the heart, and that an important coronary artery might be occluded with survival of the subject and with little or no evidence of infarction.

Gross, in 1921, confirmed Langer's studies, and stated that advanced age was a stimulus to this collateral [14]. Woodruff [15] and Wearn [16], in 1926 and 1928 respectively, demonstrated communications between the smaller branches of the coronary arterial tree, and the vasa vasorum and other vessels of the ascending aorta. In 1932, Hudson et al injected coronary ostia, showing extensive extracardiac anastomoses through the pericardiophrenic branch of the internal mammary artery, the anterior mediastinal, pericardial, bronchial, superior and inferior phrenic, intercostal and esophageal branches of the aorta [17]. The most extensive anastomoses between the cardiac and extracardiac vessels were around the ostia of the pulmonary veins, the root of the aorta, pulmonary artery, vena cavae, and at the level of the pericardial reflections. Moritz et al reported that in four patients, the extracardiac coronary anastomoses were increased when pericardial adhesions were present [18]. This formed the basis for the surgical production of pericardial adhesions to augment these extracardiac anastomoses.

Subsequent investigations confirmed these earlier findings. Roberts of Galveston [19] reported on his injection studies in dogs, which demonstrated that the Thebesian vessels could conduct blood from the left ventricle into the myocardium when the pressure in the coronary artery was lower than that in the ventricle. Paul Zoll et al, years later performed injection studies in over 1,000 randomly selected human hearts which convinced them that the coronary arteries were end arteries and collaterals developed only on stimulation [20]. Their studies showed rather common collaterals, especially in presence of coronary disease, where they felt the common denominator was relative myocardial anoxia.

Beck began his investigations by attaching a pedicle graft of pectoralis major muscle to the heart to promote the development of blood flow from the graft to the myocardium. He felt a reduced coronary blood flow to the area would promote blood flow through the pedicle, so he studied the effect of simultaneous coronary artery ligation. He was encouraged enough by the laboratory results to perform his first clinical case in 1935; one year later he had operated on eleven patients, and half of them survived [21,22].

The British surgeon, O'Shaughnessy, observed that omentum, used for certain surgical procedures, had the capacity to form new vascular adhesions [23]. He developed a series of animal experiments, using isolated greater omentum brought through the diaphragm and sutured to the surface of the heart. He performed elaborate animal experiments, including staged procedures, wherein he rendered the myocardium ischemic by ligating a coronary artery; weeks later after applying the omentum he noted a return of normal exercise performance in the animals. Ultimately the animals were sacrificed and injection studies done on the pedicle. Other tissues were used for grafting, including pericardial fat, stomach, skin, and lung. O'Shaughnessy felt so confident about his experimental data, in 1936 he performed his first omental graft procedure, and in 1937 he did cardiopneumopexy with dramatic clinical results [24]. Simultaneously other investigators, notably Reinhoff of Hopkins, were performing cardioomentopexies in dogs, and the animals were surviving subsequent coronary artery ligation [25].

Mercier Fauteux, working in Montreal and Boston, was interested in ligation of the great cardiac vein as a method of increasing myocardial blood flow [26]. He described, in the experimental animal, circulatory readjustments occurring in the coronary system after ligation of the great cardiac vein. Experimental evidence showed that great cardiac vein ligation permitted the animal to survive subsequent ligation of a coronary artery. In 1941, he described a patient operated almost two years earlier, who was now entirely free of pain. He had operated on five more patients, but the follow-up was rather short. He postulated that, in the patient with progressive arteriosclerotic narrowing of the coronary arteries, ligation of the great cardiac vein might at least limit the size of an infarct. Fauteux was also interested in pericardial neurectomy [27]. He and Ovar Swenson reported favorable results when this procedure was done alone or combined with great cardiac vein ligation [28]. By the mid-1940s he had operated on nine patients; seven were alive and well.

To perform a "cardiopericardiopexy," Beck used various substances, including such irritants as powdered beef bone, asbestos, and dilute trichloracetic acid. To enhance the formation of adhesions, he also performed epicardiectomy. In 1941, Heimbecker and Barton experimented with the use of other irritants, such as aleuronat, gelatin, starch, glycerine and water in a mixture which they instilled into the pericardial sac of dogs, using a grease gun [29]. Approximately half of the dogs so treated later survived ligation of branches of the left coronary artery.

Beck's work dominated the field. By 1941, he had abandoned the pectoralis muscle flap procedure in favor of partial occlusion of the coronary sinus, together with some method to induce adhesions between the pericardium and heart. Of these experiments, a procedure became known as the Beck I operation. This consisted of narrowing the coronary sinus to a diameter of three millimeters, abrasion of the visceral pericardium and epicardium, then adding the powdered asbestos and trichloracetic acid and mediastinal fat. This operation became very popular and was practiced extensively. In 1955, he reported with Leighninger his impressive clinical results [30]. Over 90% of patients were improved, and 50% were relieved of angina, and most had returned to work. A surgical mortality of 6.6% was felt to be due to the severity of the underlying disease. While 12% died within two years of surgery, 40% of the medically treated patients had succumbed in the same interval.

Beck worked on another procedure which he had performed as early as 1948; Roberts, in 1943, had proposed such surgery for arteriosclerotic narrowing of the coronary arteries. This operation was in two stages, and based upon the knowledge of the presence of arteriovenous communications in the myocardium. The first stage consisted of inserting an arterial graft between the thoracic aorta and the coronary sinus. In the second stage, performed a few weeks later, he surgically narrowed the coronary sinus ostium. In 1954, Beck described his results as favorable, and it became known as the Beck II operation [30, 31]. It never gained popularity, however, as it was a more complex procedure attended with a high mortality, and the lesser, or Beck I operation, had already gained a considerable amount of popularity, was safe, and with good clinical results.

Another attempt to divert mediastinal blood to the heart consisted in ligating the internal mammary artery distal to the origin of the pericardiophrenic artery. In 1939, such a procedure was performed in Italy at the suggestion of Fieschi. This operation was based on his earlier work which, with radiopaque injection, demonstrated a vascular pathway between the internal mammary artery through the pericardiophrenic branch into the periaortic and peripulmonary arterial rami. In 1955 this work was amplified by cadaver studies and dog experiments by Dr. Battezzali et al, who later operated on 25 patients with good results [32,33].

Glover et al [34], in a comprehensive paper in 1957, questioned whether these extracardiac anastomoses with the coronary artery bed were sufficient to significantly increase coronary artery blood flow. He reported an elaborate study in animals, to quantitate the blood flow when both internal mammary arteries were ligated. The results showed that there was indeed communication, and that these afforded protection to the heart when coronary arteries were ligated. Clinically he believed this procedure should be performed with cautious optimism. One distinct advantage, he felt, was the minimal surgery required to ligate an internal mammary artery -- this could be done under local anesthesia through a small incision in the left second interspace. He thought this a definite advantage over the other procedures then popular, which required general anesthetic, a thoracotomy or sternotomy. He reported upon seventy-seven patients submitted to this operation. Fifty were followed from one to five months. There was improvement in 68% of the patients, while 22% demonstrated no change. The five deaths occurred in patients who had had more than one myocardial infarction in their past history.

These seemingly positive clinical results, however, were not substantiated by further laboratory experiments. Sabiston and Blalock, in 1958, reported their results of ligating the left internal mammary artery [35]. They were specifically interested in the volume of blood that could be directed through the pericardiophrenic vessel following ligation of the ipsilateral internal mammary artery. They found, in the normal dog heart, that the volume of blood flow was small, increasing only slightly with the passage of time. They, however, noted that the flow did increase if other branches of internal mammary were ligated, such as the thyrocervical trunk. When a coronary artery was ligated as part of the procedure, they found no protective effect of ligating the internal mammary artery. Shortly thereafter, Vansant and Muller confirmed these results [36]. Few surgeons believed that internal mammary ligation was a rational approach to the problem, and most surgeons never performed it. In fact, sham operations were devised and produced the same clinical results!

Another approach to augmenting coronary collateral blood flow rose out of the observation in cyanotic congenital heart disease of the greatly increased coronary arborization. In 1959, Day and Lillehei created a pulmonary artery-to-left atrial shunt, in fact, a right-to-left shunt to produce cyanosis and increase coronary artery arborization [37]. This idea, which originated in the USSR, proved of no merit. Another attempt to increase coronary blood flow involved surgically creating an ascending aortic coarctation. This concept in theory, however, would increase systolic resistance, causing increased cardiac work and oxygen requirements.

These arduous experiments and clinical trials ultimately came to an end. Their value, however, was undisputed, as much was learned about the coronary circulation, the inter- and intracoronary collateral, and the effect of reduced blood flow on myocardial segments.

Direct Myocardial Revascularization
Confidence derived from successes in operations on some congenital cardiac lesions and acquired mitral stenosis, suggested bolder methods to treat coronary heart disease. The coronary arteries were being recognized to be of a sufficient size and appropriate location to render them suitable for direct reconstruction and bypass. Impetus for this work was derived in part from the success that surgeons were experiencing working on the larger peripheral vessels of the body using a variety of conduits including saphenous vein, plastic and homograft tissue. So experiments were devised to perform primary anastomosis between cut ends of in situ coronary arteries, as well as performing local endarterectomy of obstructing arterial segments. Knowledge concerning the nature and location of the obstructing

lesions in the coronary arteries was growing.

The decade of the 1950s witnessed much activity in techniques applied directly to the coronary arteries. Again, the procedures were carried out principally in animals, with some clinical trials thereafter. The visionary surgeon, Alexis Carrel, in the first decade of the century, conceived the idea of coronary artery bypass, and performed such an operation in dogs by interposing a segment of carotid artery between the thoracic aorta and the coronary artery [38]. But it was the innovative surgeon, Gordon Murray, of Toronto, in 1953, who did extensive experimental work in dogs, interposing venous or arterial grafts to replace stenotic coronary artery segments [39]. Interruption of blood flow in the coronary arteries during these procedures, however, caused myocardial infarcts. He then experimented with perfusion of the distal segment of the coronary artery with a variety of solutions, including oxygenated heparinized blood. Experiments were carried out using the internal mammary artery and free grafts between the subclavian artery and a coronary artery. The internal mammary artery proved too small. The first clinical effort, while unsuccessful, was performed by William Mustard, also of Toronto; he bypassed an anomalous left coronary artery using a carotid artery, under mild hypothermia [40].

In 1952, the Soviet surgeon, Demikhov, began work on anastomosis of the internal mammary artery to a coronary artery. Seven years later, one dog was alive and well. News of this important research did not reach the Western world until 1962; however, when it did, it introduced a key component of modern day coronary artery surgery [41]. By 1967, Kolessov reported experience with six patients [42].

Wangensteen and associates, in Minnesota, reported efforts to maintain blood flow during experimental coronary anastomoses [43]. Oxygenated blood in a reservoir was used to perfuse the divided coronary during systemic-coronary anastomosis. In other experiments, perfusion took the form of a synthetic tube as a shunt interposed between the aorta and the distal coronary artery. Thal performed direct suture anastomosis between the internal mammary and circumflex coronary artery; using techniques mentioned above, blood flow was maintained to the myocardium. All the animals survived the surgery; at six months, however, less than one half the anastomoses were patent. The most common findings in the occluded anastomoses were strictures and thrombosis.

Beck, as early as 1932, had performed endarterectomy of coronary arteries at autopsy. The first clinical reports of coronary artery endarterectomy were those of Charles Bailey et al, in 1956 [44]. After demonstrating the feasibility in the laboratory, he applied the technique successfully in two patients. Working through a longitudinal incision in the distal vessel, he introduced a curette-like instrument designed by one of his associates to extract the proximal atheromatous core. The vessel was then closed primarily.

Cannon and Longmire performed endarterectomy on nine patients [45]. Nevertheless, they described difficulty working on the beating heart. The hearts were "irritable" and prone to hypotension, brady-arrhythmia, and even asystole. Three of the nine patients died as a result of the surgery.

Spencer took advantage of the use of cardiopulmonary bypass and hypothermic cardiac arrest to perform coronary anastomoses in sixteen dogs [46]. The resulting quiet operative field permitted meticulous microsurgical techniques, while hypothermia afforded myocardial protection. Two-thirds of the long-term survivors had patent anastomoses and the investigators credited the optimal circumstances for these good results.

Many investigators began employing these endarterectomy techniques on patients. Senning described the use of a vein patch to optimize the diameter of the arteriotomy [47,48]. As experience accumulated, improvements in survival followed. Mortality remained high, however and encouraged search for safer methods of myocardial revascularization.

In 1959, Sones introduced selective coronary arteriography, providing for the first time precise knowledge of the location and extent of the coronary lesions, as well as a method to objectively assess postoperative results [49].

A brief period of enthusiasm occurred for endarterectomy combined with the Vineberg procedure to extend myocardial revascularization. The procedure, however, would only regain popularity sometime later, when combined with saphenous vein bypass. In addition to direct endarterectomy, gas endarterectomy was introduced [50].

The first aortocoronary bypass using saphenous vein was performed by Sabiston in 1962 [51]. The procedure was unsuccessful, as the patient succumbed to a stroke. Two years later Garrett performed the first successful saphenous vein bypass as a substitute for left anterior descending coronary endarterectomy, when he encountered technical difficulties [52]. By the late 1960's, techniques were well established and safe, and, encouraged and guided by the reliability of coronary angiography, Effler and Favaloro aggressively worked on the clinical application of coronary bypass and demonstrated its effectiveness [53-55]. Meyer et al in 1968, reported on the use of the subclavian artery for bypass on an anomalous left coronary artery in a child, thereby restoring a two coronary artery system [56]. Concurrently, Spencer and Green [57] were gaining experience using the left internal mammary artery as a bypass conduit. The modern era of myocardial revascularization had begun.

Acknowledgment

The author gratefully acknowledges the editorial assistance of Margaret W. Stevenson in the preparation of this manuscript.

References

1. Heberden W. Commentaries on the History and Cure of Diseases. (Facsimile of the 1802 edition). New York Academy of Medicine, 1962; Hafner pp 361-9.
2. Herrick JB. Clinical features of sudden occlusion of the coronary arteries. JAMA 1912; 59:2015-20.
3. Harken AH. The very beginning. In: Stephenson LW, Ruggiero R: Heart Surgery Classics. Boston, 1994; Adams Publishing Group Ltd., pp 4-5.
4. Franck Francois CE: Signification physiologique de la resection du sympathetique dans le maladie de Basedow, l'epilepsie, l'idiotie et le glaucome. Bull Acad Med Paris 1899; 41:565-94.
5. Jonnesco T. Angine de poitrine guerie par le resection du sympathique cervicothoracic. Bull Acad de Med 1920; 84:93-102.
6. Coffey WB, Brown PK. Surgical treatment of angina pectoris. Arch Int Med 1923; 31:200-220.
7. Cutler EC. Summary of experiences up-to-date in the surgical treatment of angina pectoris. Am J Med Sci 1927; 173:613-24.
8. Blumgart HL, Levine SA, Berlin DD. Congestive heart failure and angina pectoris. The therapeutic effect of thyroidectomy on patients without clinical and pathologic evidence of thyroid toxicity. Arch Int Med 1933; 51:866-77.
9. Blumgart HL, Riseman JEF, Davis D, Berlin DD. Therapeutic effect of total ablation of normal thyroid on congestive heart failure and angina pectoris. III. Early results in various types of cardiovascular disease and coincident pathologic states without clinical or pathologic evidence of thyroid toxicity. Arch Int Med 1933; 52:165-225.
10. Cutler EC, Levine SA. La douleur angineuse et son traitement chirurgical. Valeur des differentes methodes, et plus particoulierement de la thyroidectomie totale. Presse Med 1934; 46:937-40.
11. Braunwald E, Sonnenblick EH, Frommer PL, et al. Paired electric stimulation of the heart: physiologic observations and clinical implications. Adv Int Med 1967; 13:61-96.
12. Beck CS, Tichy VL. Production of collateral circulation to heart; experimental study. Am Heart J 1935; 10:849-873.
13. Langer L. Die Foramina Thebesii in Herzen des Menschen. Sitzungsb, d.k. Akad. Wissensch, Math-Naturw, 1880; 82:3, Abth 1880; 25-39.
14. Gross L, Blum L, Silverman G. Experimental attempts to increase the blood supply to the dog's heart by means of coronary sinus occlusion. J Exper Med 1937; 65:91-108.
15. Woodruff EC. Studies on the vasa vasorum. Am J Pathol 1926; 2:568.
16. Wearn JT. The extent of the capillary bed of the heart. J Exper Med 1928; 47:273.
17. Hudson C, Moritz A, Wearn JT. The extracardiac anastomoses of the coronary arteries. J Exper Med 1932; 56:919-25.
18. Moritz AR, Hudson CL, Orgain S. Augmentation of the extracardiac anastomoses

of the coronary arteries through pericardial adhesions. J Exper Med 1932; 56:927-31.

19. Roberts JT. Experimental studies on the nourishment of the left ventricle by the luminal (Thebesial) vessels. Fed Proc 1943; 2:90.

20. Zoll PM, Wessler S, Schlesinger MJ. Intraarterial anastomoses in the human heart, with particular reference to anemia and relative cardiac anoxia. Circulation 1951; 4:797-815.

21. Beck CS. The development of a new blood supply to the heart by operation. Ann Surg 1935; 102:801-13.

22. Beck CS. Further data on the establishment of a new blood supply to the heart by operation. J Thorac Surg 1936; 5:604-11.

23. O'Shaughnessy L. An experimental method of providing a collateral circulation to the heart. Brit J Surg 1936; 23:665-70.

24. O'Shaughnessy L. The surgery of the heart. Practitioner 1938; 140:603-18.

25. Reinhoff W. Approaches to the management of myocardial ischemia. In: Schumacher HB: The Evolution of Cardiac Surgery. Bloomington, 1992; Indiana University Press, p. 134.

26. Fauteux M, Palmer JH. Treatment of angina pectoris of atheromatous origin by ligation of the great cardiac vein. Can Med Assoc J 1941; 45:295-8 .

27. Fauteux M: Surgical treatment of angina pectoris. Experience with ligation of the great cardiac vein and pericoronary neurectomy. Ann Surg 1946; 124:1041-6.

28. Fauteux M, Swenson A. Pericoronary neurectomy in abolishing anginal pain in coronary disease. An experimental evaluation. Arch Surg 1946; 53:169-81.

29. Heimbecker P, Barton WA. An effective method for the development of collateral circulation to the myocardium. Am Surg 1941; 114:186-90.

30. Beck CS, Leighninger DS. Scientific basis of the surgical treatment of coronary artery disease. JAMA 1955; 159:1264-71.

31. Beck CS, Leighninger DS. Operations for coronary artery disease. JAMA 1954; 156:1226-33.

32. Zoja and Cesa-Bianchi: Cited In: Kitchell JR, Glover RP, Kyle RH. Bilateral internal mammary artery ligation for angina pectoris: preliminary clinical considerations. Am J Cardiol 1958; 1:46-50.

33. Battezzali M, Tagliaferro A, De Marchi G. La ligatura della due arterie mammarie interne nei disturbi di vascolarezzazione relative al prima dati speimentali e clinici. Minerva Med 1955; 46:1178-88.

34. Glover RP, Davila JC, Kyle RH, Beard JC Jr, Trout RG, Kitchell JR. Ligation of the internal mammary arteries as a means of increasing blood supply to the myocardium. J Thorac Surg 1957; 34:661-78.

35. Sabiston DC Jr, Blalock A. Experimental ligation of the internal mammary artery and its effect on coronary occlusion. Surgery 1958; 43:906-12.

36. Vansant JH, Muller WH Jr. Experimental evaluation of internal mammary artery ligation as a method of myocardial revascularization. Surgery 1959; 45:840-7.

37. Day SB, Lillehei CW. Experimental basis for a new operation for coronary artery disease; a left atrial-pulmonary artery shunt to encourage the development of

interarterial intercoronary anastomoses. Surgery 1959; 45:487.

38. Edwards WS, Edwards PD. Alexis Carrel, Visionary Surgeon. 1974, Springfield Ill, Charles C Thomas, pp 47.

39. Murray G, Porcheron R, Hilario J, Roschau W. Anastomosis of a systemic artery to the coronary. Can Med Assoc J 1954; 71:594-7.

40. Shumacher HB. The Evolution of Cardiac Surgery. Bloomington, 1992; Indiana University Press. p. 140.

41. Demikhov VP. Experimental Transplantation of Vital Organs. Authorized translation from the Russian by Basil Haigh. New York: 1962; Consultants Bureau.

42. Kolessov VI. Mammary artery-coronary artery anastomosis as method of treatment for angina pectoris. J Thorac Cardiovasc Surg 1967; 54:535-44.

43. Thal A, Perry JF Jr, Miller FA, Wangensteen OH. Direct suture anastomosis of the coronary arteries in dogs. Surgery 1956; 40:1023-9.

44. Bailey CP, May A, Lemmon WM. Survival after coronary endarterectomy in man. JAMA 1957; 164:641-6.

45. Cannon JA, Longmire WP Jr, Kattus AA. Considerations of the rationale and technique of coronary endarterectomy for angina pectoris. Surgery 1959; 46:197-211.

46. Spencer FC, Yong NK, Prachuabmoh K. Internal mammary-coronary artery anastomoses performed during cardiopulmonary bypass. J Cardiovasc Surg 1964; 5:292-7.

47. Absolon KB, Aust JB, Varco RL, Lillehei CW. Surgical treatment of occlusive coronary artery disease by endarterectomy or anastomotic replacement. Surg Gynec Obst 1956; 103:180-5.

48. Effler DB, Groves LK, Sones FM Jr, Shirey EK. Endarterectomy in the treatment of coronary artery disease. J Thorac Cardiovasc Surg 1964; 47:98-108.

49. Sones FM, Shirey EK. Cinecoronary arteriography. Mod Concepts Cardiovasc Dis 1962; 31:735-8.

50. Sawyer PN, Kaplitt M, Sobel S, et al. Experimental and clinical experience with gas endarterectomy. Arch Surg 1967; 95:736-42.

51. Sabiston DC Jr. Direct surgical management of congenital and acquired lesions of the coronary artery. Prog Cardiovasc Dis 1963; 6:299-316.

52. Garrett HE, Dennis EW, DeBakey ME. Aortocoronary bypass with saphenous vein graft. Seven-year followup. JAMA 1973; 223:792-4.

53. Favaloro RG. Saphenous vein autograft replacement of severe segmental coronary artery occlusion. Ann Thorac Surg 1968; 5:334-9.

54. Favaloro RG. Saphenous vein graft in the surgical treatment of coronary artery disease. Operative technique. J Thorac Cardiovasc Surg 1969; 58:178-85.

55. Favaloro RG, Effler DB, Groves LK, Sheldon WC, Riahi M. Direct myocardial revascularization with saphenous vein autograft. Clinical experience with 100 cases. Dis Chest 1969; 56:279-83.

56. Meyer BW, Stefanik G, Stiles QR, Lindesmith GG, Jones JC. A method of definitive treatment of anomalous origin of left coronary artery. A case report. J Thorac Cardiovasc Surg 1968; 56:104-7.

57. Spencer FC, Green GE, Tice DA, Glassman E. Surgical therapy for coronary artery disease. Curr Probl Surg Sept, 1970.

Additional References of Historical Interest

Absolon KB, Mispireta LA. The past, present and future of the surgical treatment of atherosclerotic heart disease. Rev Surg 1975; 32:1-21.

Baltaxe HA, Amplatz K, Levin DC. Coronary Angiography. Springfield, Illinois, 1973, Charles C Thomas.

Beck CS, Leighninger DS. Operations for coronary artery disease. JAMA 1954; 156:1226-33.

Bing RJ (editor): Cardiology. The Evolution of the Science and the Art. Philadelphia, 1992, Harwood Academic Publishers.

Blumgart HL, Schlesinger MJ, Davis D. Studies on relation of clinical manifestation of angina pectoris, coronary thrombosis and myocardial infarction to pathologic findings, with particular reference to significance of collateral circulation. Am Heart J 1940; 19:1-91.

Effler DB, Sones FM Jr, Favaloro RF, Groves LK. Coronary endarterectomy with patch-graft reconstruction. Clinical experience with 34 cases. Ann Surg 1965; 162:590-601.

Garrett EH, Dennis EW, DeBakey ME. Aortocoronary bypass with saphenous vein grafts. Seven-year follow-up. JAMA 1973; 223:792-4.

Gensini GG. Coronary Arteriography, 1975, Mount Kisco New York, Futura Publishing Company.

Goetz RH, Rohman M, Haller JD, et al. Internal mammary-coronary artery anastomosis -- a nonsuture method employing tantalum rings. J Thorac Cardiovasc Surg 1961; 41:378-86.

Johnson WD, Flemma RJ, Lepley D Jr, Ellison EH. Extended treatment of severe coronary artery disease: a total surgical approach. Ann Surg 1969;170:460-70.

Mayo CH: Discussion: Lilienthal H. Cervical sympathectomy in angina. A report of three cases. Arch Surg 1925; 10:531-43.

Ochsner JL, Mills NL. Coronary Artery Surgery. Philadelphia, 1978, Lea & Febiger.

Rosenblum HH, Levine SA. What happens eventually to patients with hyperthyroidism and significant heart disease following subtotal thyroidectomy. Am J Med Sci 1933; 185:219-33.

Segall HN. Pioneers of Cardiology in Canada, 1820-1970. Willowdale, Ontario, Canada, 1988, Hounslow Press.

Stiles QR, Tucker BL, Lindesmith GG, Meyer BW. Myocardial Revascularization, a Surgical Atlas. Boston, 1976, Little Brown & Co.

White JC. Cardiac pain. Anatomic pathways and physiologic mechanisms. Circulation, 1957; 16:644-55.

2

THE VINEBERG PROCEDURE IN THE ERA OF TRANSMYOCARDIAL REVASCULARIZATION
A New Paradigm for an Old Operation

John C. Tsang, Carlos M. Li, Ray C.-J. Chiu
The Division of Cardiovascular & Thoracic Surgery, McGill University, Montréal, Quebec, Canada.

Dr. Arthur Vineberg was born in Montreal, on May 24, 1903. He was trained at McGill University and received his M.D. and M.Sc. degrees in 1928. He completed his residency and also obtained a Ph.D in experimental surgery in 1933. He was an attending staff at the Royal Victoria Hospital from 1935 to 1965, served as chief of the division of cardiac surgery from 1956 to 1965 and was an associate professor of surgery at McGill University. He published over 250 articles and three books. Dr. Vineberg died on March 26, 1988.

18 Direct Myocardial Revascularization

INTRODUCTION

The Vineberg procedure consists of implanting the internal mammary artery (IMA) directly into an area of ischemic myocardium. The principle behind its success, as described by Dr. Vineberg, is that the implanted artery will develop communications with the "sinusoidal" system within the myocardium, allowing a delivery system of nutrients to ischemic areas which cannot be supplied by occluded epicardial coronary arteries. This was one of the first widely adopted surgical options for treatment of ischemic heart disease and over 15,000 IMA implants had been performed up until the 1970's. However, skepticism of its physiological basis and the popularization of direct coronary revascularization by Favoloro, led to the abandonment of the Vineberg procedure.

Recently, interest has surged on the use of transmyocardial laser revascularization (TMR) in patients with non-bypassable coronary artery disease. The original concept for TMR is that the transmural channels created by laser would allow communications between the ventricular cavity and the myocardial sinusoids to provide nutrient flow. With interest growing in this patient population of "terminal vessel disease" and the fact that the proposed mechanism for TMR is similar to that originally proposed by Vineberg for his operation, it is time to review the Vineberg procedure and its possible role in the era of TMR.

Extensive accounts on the historical development of the Vineberg procedure are available. For an excellent recent review the reader is referred to the article by Shrager [1]. This chapter will instead attempt to reassess the Vineberg procedure and its underlying concepts in light of more recent advances in myocardial revascularization.

THE OPERATION AND EXPERIMENTAL VALIDATION

Dr. Vineberg originally described his technique of myocardial revascularization in 1946 [2]. Through a left thoracotomy, the fifth intercostal space was entered, the internal mammary artery was freed from the chest wall between the 4th and 6th costal cartilage (Figure 1; from reference 4 (p.72)). With the heart still beating, the epicardium was incised at two sites separated by about 2 cm. The IMA was then tunneled through the myocardium between the two incisions, with its distal end ligated but with the 6th intercostal artery branch left open and allowed to bleed into the myocardium (Figure 2; from reference 4 (p. 73)).

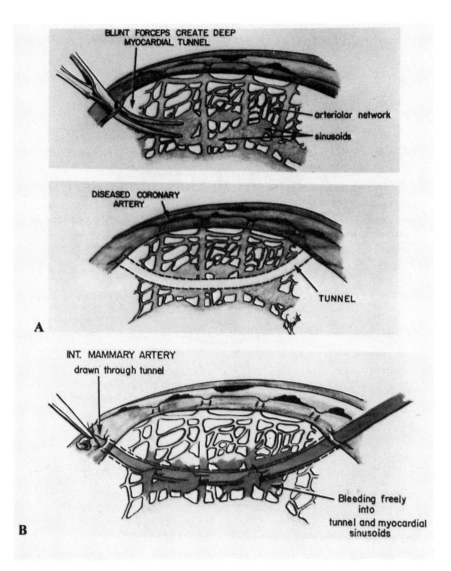

Figure 1. Vineberg's technique of IMA implantation (Reprinted with permission of the publisher from Vineberg AM. Myocardial Revascularization by Arterial/Ventricular Implants, p. 72. Massachusetts, John Wright/PSG Inc, 1982).

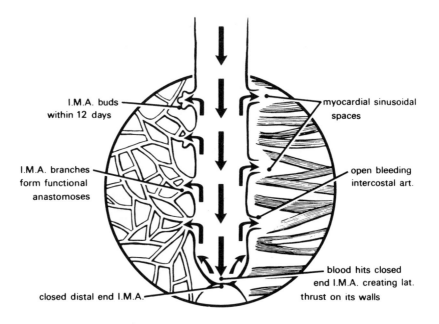

I.M.A. buds within 12 days

myocardial sinusoidal spaces

I.M.A. branches form functional anastomoses

open bleeding intercostal art.

blood hits closed end I.M.A. creating lat. thrust on its walls

closed distal end I.M.A.

Figure 2. Vineberg's conceptualization of the factors which maintain IMA implant patency and formation of implant to coronary anastomoses (Reprinted with permission of the publisher from Vineberg AM. Myocardial Revascularization by Arterial/Ventricular Implants, p. 73. Massachusetts, John Wright/PSG Inc, 1982).

Vineberg performed the first clinical IMA implantation in 1950. The first patient died a few days after surgery, but the next two patients survived [3].

Vineberg reviewed injection studies of the heart, autopsy specimens and angiographic patterns of the branching and terminations of the coronary circulation to determine the optimal locations for IMA implantation. These so called "triarteriolar zones" in the left ventricular apex, anterolateral and anterobasal walls, were the areas of the terminations of the left anterior descending, circumflex, and right coronary arteries and/or their branches (Figure 3; from reference 4 (p.260-262)). He proposed that when properly performed, an implant inserted into these

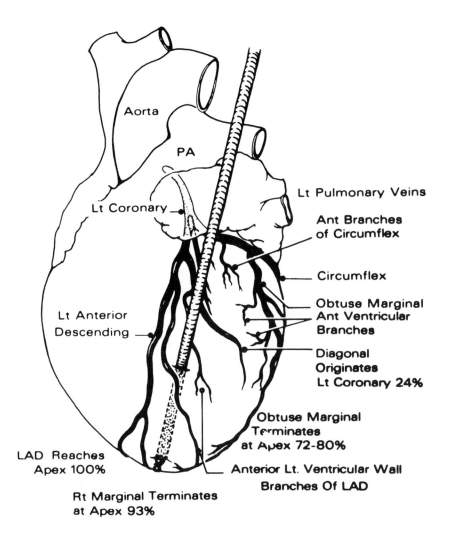

Figure 3. "Triarteriolar" implantation sites of the left ventricle: a) Apical
(Reprinted with permission of the publisher from Vineberg AM. Myocardial
Revascularization by Arterial/Ventricular Implants, p. 260-262. Massachusetts,
John Wright/PSG Inc, 1982).

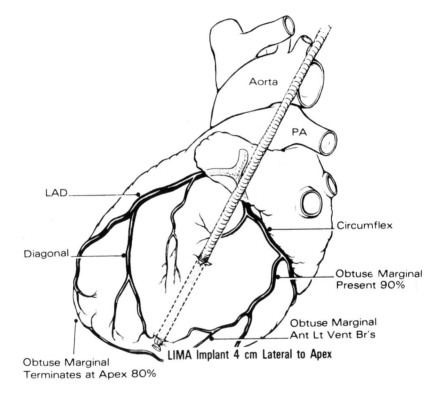

Figure 3. (b) Anterolateral implantation site.

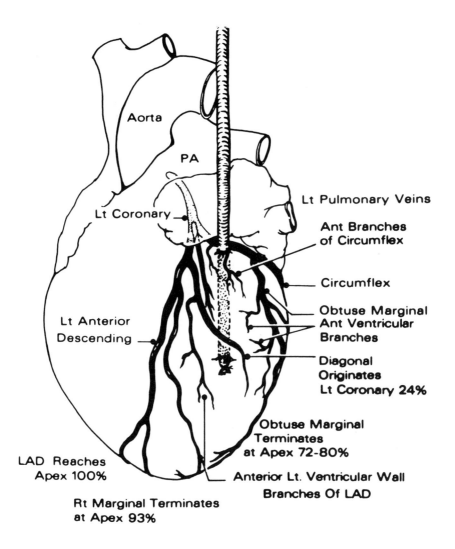

Figure 3. (c) Anterobasal implantation site.

critical zones would be able to provide new circulation to the territory supplied by the respective occluded surface coronaries [4, 57].

Extensive experimental and clinical work was presented by Vineberg supporting the beneficial function of the implanted IMA. In his initial paper, Vineberg showed by injection of Schlesinger solution into an IMA implant four months post-op, the injectate could be seen in the coronaries and the aorta. He proposed that the injected solution "obviously reached the aorta through the coronary orifice" and that this occurred because of the development of an IMA to coronary anastomosis [2]. Another early study was done using a dog model of chronic ischemia, induced by wrapping the left anterior descending artery in cellophane to cause sclerosis. Vineberg showed that exercise tolerance of the dogs would gradually improve three to five months after IMA implant surgery, from 1.6 minutes to 6-8 minutes. This was again attributed to the development of IMA to coronary anastomosis and, as well, demonstrated the functional value of such anastomoses [5, 6]. Subsequently, other investigators such as Reis confirmed the benefit of the procedure by demonstrating preservation of ventricular function in an ischemic model with IMA implants. In dogs, Reis showed that after IMA implantation and coronary ligation, preservation of ventricular function was dependent on a patent IMA implant (Figure 4; [9]).

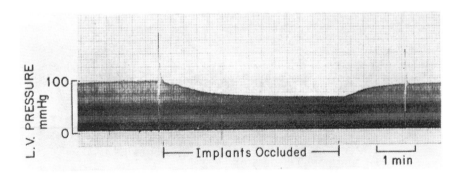

Figure 4. Experimental occlusion of a functioning IMA implant in a dog with resultant depression in ventricular function and subsequent recovery. (From Reis RL et al. Ann Surg 1970;171:9-16 with permission).

Despite proper implantation into Vineberg's so called "triarteriolar zones", the beneficial effects of the implants did not occur immediately but only after six weeks to six months [10, 11, 34]. Therefore for the sicker patients who required immediate revascularization, Vineberg augmented the IMA implant with additional procedures to provide an immediate source of blood supply. He advocated epicardiectomy and the Ivalon sponge procedures to this end. The epicardiectomy was done so that external supply of blood from the pericardium and mediastinum could be brought to the myocardium, and the Ivalon sponge would act as a framework along which the blood vessels could grow [12]. This blood supply would then enter the "sponge-like" myocardium and communicate with the network of arterioluminal vessels first described by Wearn [13], so that ventricular blood could enter the arterioluminal and arteriorsinusoidal space (Figure 5; reference 4 (p.16)). Vineberg felt that this would bring an immediate source of blood supply, "within an hour" to the ischemic myocardium and bridge the patient until the IMA implant was fully functional. The evidence of the effectiveness of these additional procedures was demonstrated by injection studies of explanted hearts which had been treated with epicardiectomy and the Ivalon sponge. The Schlesinger mass injected into the left ventricular lumen would appear in the distal coronary arteries suggesting that there was ventricular luminal to myocardial flow [14]. Subsequently, the use of the Ivalon sponge was abandoned because of its carcinogenicity. However, the epicardiectomy itself was thought to "open(ed) up the 400 million year old arterioluminal vessels, luminal sinusoidal vessels and myocardial sinusoidal spaces within the myocardium" [13]. A further adjunct to enhance early revascularization in the IMA implants was the use of free omental grafting. Vineberg felt that the omentum had an inherent ability to stimulate new collaterals from the pericardium and mediastinum. He attempted to demonstrate this via various injection experiments and pathological studies [15, 16]. The use of these additional procedures of epicardiectomy, Ivalon sponge and free omental graft, due to their lack of scientific validation, compromised the acceptance of Vineberg's ideas in the eyes of the medical community. Finally, Vineberg introduced one final element into his arsenal, the right ventricular IMA implant. He noted that several patients returned with recurrent angina despite functioning left ventricular implants. These patients all had right coronary occlusions. Thus, he added right IMA implants to the left IMA implants. The right IMA to right ventricular implants worked differently from the left ventricular implants in that the latter were felt to have flow mainly during diastole, as in the coronary circulation, while right ventricular implants provided constant flow because the systemic pressures throughout each cardiac cycle was greater than the maximal right ventricular pressure [10]. In addition, because the sinusoidal spaces of the right

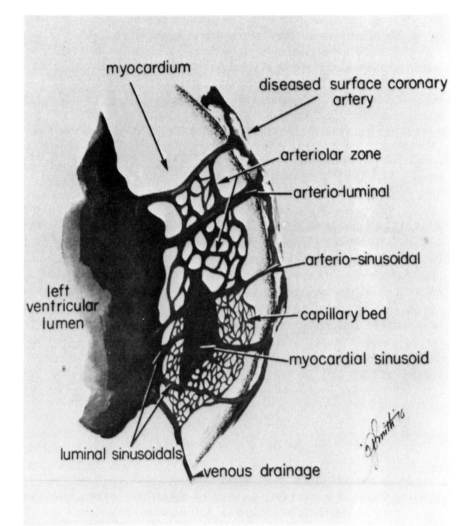

Figure 5. Artist's rendition of the concept of sinusoids (Reprinted with permission of the publisher from Vineberg AM. Myocardial Revascularization by Arterial/Ventricular Implants, p.16. Massachusetts, John Wright/PSG Inc, 1982).

ventricle were in continuity with those of the left ventricle, the RV implants were felt to also improve left ventricular ischemia [17]. This concept was again assessed via injection, and digestion cast studies. Thus, armed with his four part procedure of epicardiectomy, free omental graft, and bilateral IMA implant, Vineberg took on patients with severe two or three vessel disease.

PATHOPHYSIOLOGY: OLD PARADIGM AND CHALLENGES

Vineberg's rationale for his procedure was based on the concept of the myocardial sinusoids described by Wearn in the 1930's [13]. The belief was that a bleeding artery could be implanted within the inner third of the myocardium (as this would allow for the optimal pressure gradient) without thrombosis of the IMA and resultant obliteration of the artery because the myocardium consisted of a sponge like network of sinusoids [18]. These sinusoids were thought to be an endothelial lined network of interconnecting potential space which would provide adequate run-off to maintain implant patency. The effect was enhanced when the IMA was implanted into an area of hypoperfusion, encouraging anastomoses with the nearby occluded coronaries [19]. Vineberg tested his hypothesis in models of chronic coronary ischemia created by the use of ameroid constrictors which gradually caused fibrosis of the coronary [20]. His experimental and clinical studies in support of his hypothesis often used injection of vinyl acetate and digestion casts of implanted hearts to demonstrate these sponge like myocardial sinusoids [8, 10, 17] (Figure 6; reference 4(p.129)). Histological sections of explanted implant specimens were also felt to demonstrate evidence of growth of new collaterals (> 40 μm) between the implants and the native circulation [7]. His conceptual paradigm was however contested by others in the early 1970's.

Work by Chiu questioned the validity of sinusoids as an explanation for the functionality of the Vineberg procedure [21]. In a dog model, intra-myocardial IMA implantation was performed. A colloidal suspension of India ink was infused through the IMA, and distribution was found to be mainly within the interstitial space (Figure 7; [21]). Using nucleated chicken blood as a marker, it was demonstrated that very few red cells coming from the implant entered the coronary vasculature with most cells ending up in interstitial space (Figure 8; [21]). The early flow through the IMA was minimal at physiological pressures. The question was, if the blood flow through the IMA was minimal, why was the IMA implant patency rate reported in the literature high?

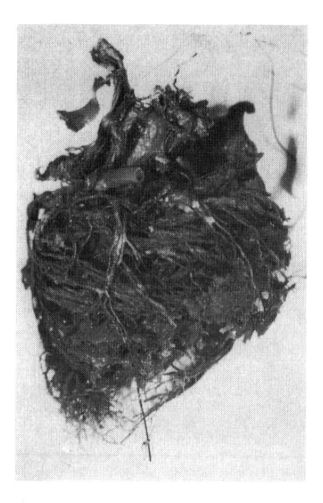

Figure 6. Vinyl-acetate cast of a ventricular implant depicting the so-called sinusoidal spaces arranged in palisades. (Reprinted with permission of the publisher from Vineberg AM. Myocardial Revascularization by Arterial/ Ventricular Implants, p. 129. Massachusetts, John Wright/PSG Inc, 1982).

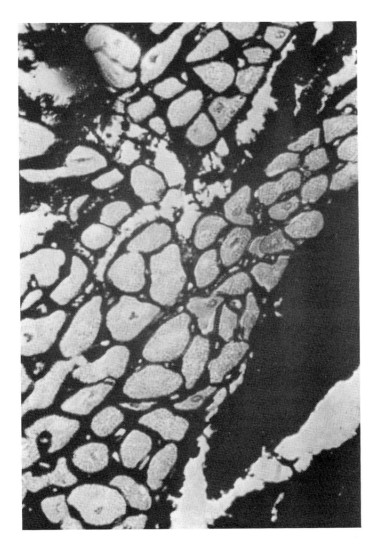

Figure 7. Colloid suspension infused through an IMA implant found predominantly in the interstitial space (From Chiu CJ et al. J Thorac and Cardiovasc Surg 1973;65:768-777 with permission).

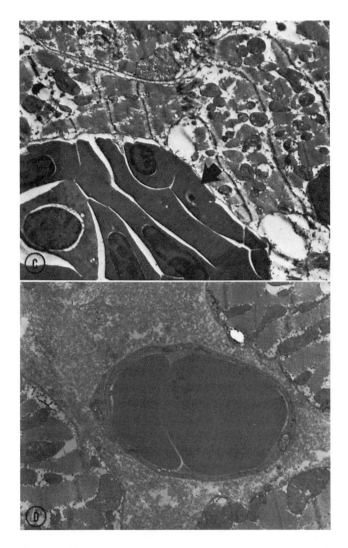

Figure 8. Electron microscopic view demonstrating that the nucleated avian erythrocytes infused through the myocardial implant are directly adjacent to the sarcolemma of the muscle fiber without intervening endothelium; whereas the anucleated canine erythrocytes from the coronary circulation are found within the endothelium-lined capillary. (From Chiu CJ et al. J Thorac and Cardiovasc Surg 1973;65:768-777 with permission).

Carlson attempted to answer this issue of IMA implant patency in spite of low flow. In a dog model, varying length of either the IMA or vein graft were implanted into the myocardium. It was noted that vessels implanted for a significant length (6-11 cm) had the most phasic to-and-fro flow and nearly 100% patency rate at 48 hours. This was in contrast to vessels minimally or not implanted into the myocardium, where phasic flow was minimal or absent, and high incidence of thrombosis of the vessels was noted. Fibrinogen content was noted to be significantly reduced in the buried segment and it correlated with the magnitude of phasic flow [22].

Baird attempted to decipher the real mechanism of success in the Vineberg procedure [23]. With the accumulating evidence, Baird did not believe in the concept of myocardial sinusoids as the reason the IMA implants remained patent and proposed an alternate hypothesis. At initial implant, the forward flow was nearly zero through the graft. Patency was maintained by the concept proposed by Carlson of to-and-fro flow and defibrination of intraluminal blood of the implant. Connections between the IMA and the coronary system would develop as a consequence of granulation tissue developing in the implant tunnel (Figure 9; from reference [58]). Enlargement of these collaterals into functionally significant IMA-coronary collaterals was dependent upon three sources of positive pressure gradient. First, the gradient between the IMA and coronary artery due to the phasic delay of the pulse wave in the IMA, allowing a positive gradient to occur in late systole and early diastole (Figure 10; from reference [59]). Second, a positive gradient developed if the IMA was implanted in a location supplied by a stenotic coronary artery with "hypotensive" perfusion pressures. Third, a positive pressure gradient was generated dependent upon the design of the tunnel. Specifically, by the nature of the tunneling method, the middle third of the tunnel was deeper and closer to the endocardium than the proximal and distal third (Figure 11). Due to the intramyocardial pressures, the blood in the middle third of the implant was subjected to the highest intramyocardial during isovolumetric contraction and ejection phase of systole. As a result, blood in the distal third of the IMA was trapped and compressed with resultant pressures of 60-80 mm Hg greater than aortic pressures. This initial compression of the deepest middle third of the IMA resulted in the so called "systolic wink", evident on some post-implant angiograms, and was felt to further promote the development of collaterals to nearby occluded coronaries.

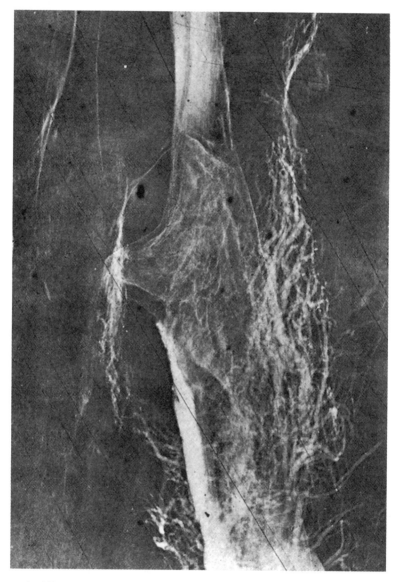

Figure 9. Microangiograph from an autopsy specimen shows an IMA implant surrounded by newly formed capillaries. (From Trapp WG et al. J Thorac Cardiovasc Surg 1969;57:451).

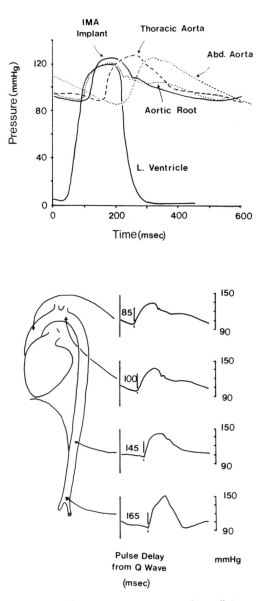

Figure 10. Phasic delay of the pulse contour at various distances from the aortic valve as demonstrated by superimposed pressure tracings. (Modified from Baird RJ et al Ann Surg 1968;168:736-749).

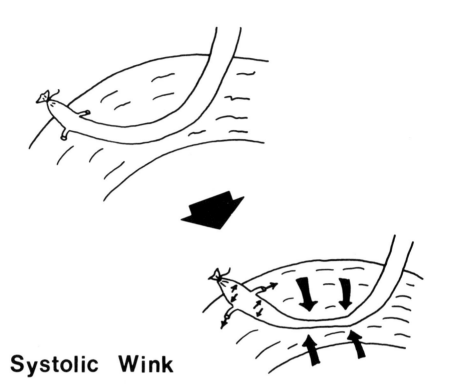

Systolic Wink

Figure 11. Diagram depicting the effect of tunneling the middle third of the implant towards the deepest aspect of the myocardium, creating the "systolic wink" phenomena.

Although Vineberg's original concept of sinusoidal flow for his procedure was not born out by experimental work, it appeared that some patients did benefit from the operation. Vineberg's original laboratory experiments where dogs after the IMA implantation showed dependency on this graft for myocardial function [5, 6, 24] was corroborated with multiple anecdotal clinical cases which followed [3, 8, 25, 26]. Many clinical studies (although few had randomized controls [27]) were performed in an attempt to validate the benefit of this operation [11, 28-31].

CLINICAL RESULTS

The clinical evidence of efficacy for the Vineberg procedure remained inconclusive. Initially, prior to the development of Sones technique for coronary arteriogram [32], much of the evidence was based on the clinical evaluation of patients and post-mortem studies. The initial clinical series was reported by Vineberg in 1954, where he reported follow-up of three years in twelve patients [33]. Nine patients had stable angina, while three had unstable angina. Of the patients with stable angina, there were no perioperative deaths, and 8 of 9 had clinical improvement (89%). The 3 patients with unstable angina died in the perioperative period. Autopsy of the first patient revealed a patent IMA, with a fresh thrombus in the circumflex, and a previous complete occlusion of the left anterior descending artery. In his second report, Vineberg reported similar results in 45 patients [34]. Perioperative mortality was 6% for patients with Class 2 or 3 angina, while those with unstable Class 4 angina had a 40-50% mortality. Nearly 80% showed symptomatic improvement. Vineberg emphasized that collateral development between the IMA and coronary arterial system required six weeks to two months as observed in his experimental studies. Therefore, he believed that patients with severe Class 4 disease required a more immediate revascularization provided by his adjuncts of epicardiectomy and free omental graft and even conventional aorto-coronary vein bypass grafts.

Implant patency has been reported as between 50-85% with double implants having better patency rates [26-29, 31, 35]. Ochsner et al noted that in patients with severe three vessel disease, there seemed to be a good correlation between implant patency and relief of symptoms [36]. However, Dart and colleagues as well as others found no correlation between the relief of angina and implant patency [30, 37]. Flow in the implants was demonstrated by Begg et al with scintigraphy especially for implants placed in ischemic areas [38]. Case and associates along with other investigators showed that IMA implants would increase collateral flow only when implanted into a region that had high grade arterial stenosis (75-100%) and that already developed these collateral vessels [36, 39, 40]. Vineberg believed that the long-term survival of patients was increased by the procedure and quoted many anecdotal cases of long-term survivors [26]. However, despite finding similar five year survivals to Ochsner [36] and Sewells' [41] studies, Bhayana et al [27], who published the only randomized trial (although with small numbers) of medical therapy versus Vineberg implant procedure, reported no difference in survival at ten years.

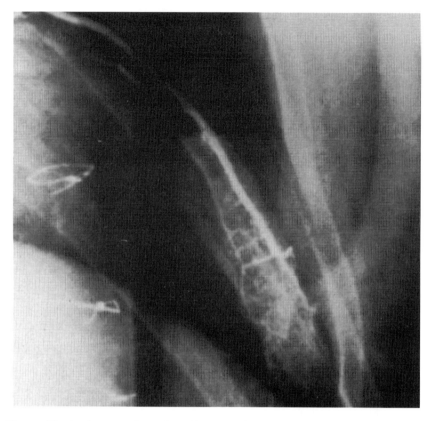

Figure 12. Angiogram of a patient 20 years after double IMA implantation for coronary occlusive disease. This view demonstrates a patent left internal mammary artery with extensive collaterals prior to reconstituting the distal anterior descending artery. (From Hayward RH et al. Ann Thorac Surg 1991;51:1002-1003 with permission)

Long-term follow-up of IMA implants (greater than twenty years) have been reported on the survival, patency and revascularization of the myocardium as demonstrated by angiographic evidence [42-44] (Figure 12; from reference [42]. There have been reports of patients who required re-operations whose hearts could not be arrested until the IMA implant was occluded [45], or that the heart fibrillated when the graft was transected, suggesting the importance of collateralization of flow from the implant to the myocardium. In a recent report, a twenty-three year old Vineberg IMA implant was shown to still provide reasonable flow to collateralized coronaries. The flow measured by Doppler echocardiography was found to be 70% that of a directly anastomosed IMA graft and that the flow reserve could reach 1.6 times basal flow as opposed to 2.6 times for a directly anastomosed graft (Figure 13; from reference [46]).

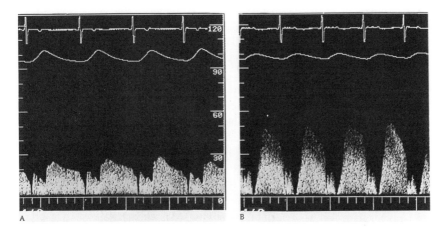

Figure 13. Doppler echocardiography demonstrating the flow reserve of a 23 year old IMA implant after administration of intravenous dipyridamole. (From Nasu M et al Ann Thor Surg 1996;61:1242-1244 with permission).

A NEW PROBLEM

The Vineberg procedure lost its appeal because of the advent of direct arterial revascularization with bypass grafts. Coronary artery bypass grafting (CABG) allowed for an immediate revascularization which was predictable as opposed to the Vineberg operation where a delay period of nearly two months was required for the development of collaterals, with results which were often unpredictable. During the late 1970's to the present, reports on the Vineberg in the literature were sparse, as the tide turned to the CABG operation. However, as the CABG operation established itself, subgroups of patients appeared that had diffuse coronary artery disease not amenable to direct revascularization. The proportion of patients with diffuse disease has been estimated to be between 8% to nearly 25% [47]. The approach for managing many of these patients has been to perform coronary endarterectomy with patch augmentation [47]. Vineberg was aware of this group and made special emphasis to the existence of this population. It was Vineberg's contention that IMA implant was a superior technique to direct coronary revascularization because of the diffuse nature of coronary atherosclerosis as opposed to the myocardial microcirculation which was relatively unaffected [10].

THE NEW PARADIGM

The development of laser transmyocardial revascularization has led to the re-introduction of the concept of "myocardial sinusoids". The original concept was that channels created with the laser would allow immediate communication between the ventricular lumen and the myocardial sinusoids, which would result in nutritive flow to the ischemic area [48]. However, much controversy has arisen regarding the role of these channels and whether they remain patent [49, 50, 51]. In addition, the presence of myocardial sinusoids has never been objectively proven and is still based on a concept described in a 1930's paper, and perpetuated by Vineberg as the rationale for his procedure. The angiographic evidence of the implants' patency and collateralization to the coronary circulation has been taken to imply the existence of sinusoidal network by default [52].

With the existence of myocardial sinusoids in question, alternative mechanisms of action have been proposed for TMR which may equally apply to the Vineberg procedure. One such hypothesis is the stimulation of angiogenesis which Vineberg himself alluded to in his book [4; p. 106]. Recently, investigators have suggested that the laser channels may in fact serve as a trigger event for the development of collateral vessels due to capillary ingrowth from an inflammatory response [53], much as the collaterals that were noted in many of the Vineberg's histological specimens which he and others had shown to develop into true arterioles of at least 40 microns in diameter [7]. Experimental studies have shown that when an IMA implant procedure is supplemented with platelet derived growth factor, there is stimulation of collateral development to an ischemic area which can protect the myocardium during acute ischemia [54]. The gradual time course of improvement of symptoms in patients who have undergone Vineberg IMA implants or TMR [55] is consistent with the concept of angiogenesis rather than the immediate benefit one would expect if the new blood flow were directed into the myocardial sinusoids. It has been similarly suggested that patients with severe heart failure are poor candidates for TMR due to the high risk of the procedure and delayed effects [56]. This is similar to Vineberg's initial concern that Class IV patients were not good candidates for the IMA implantation due to the high mortality and need for immediate revascularization which was not feasible with his operation [33].

FUTURE PERSPECTIVE

The Vineberg procedure was truly the first significant surgical therapy for ischemic heart disease. It was a procedure that has been shown to be often effective, even though probably not for the reasons Vineberg originally based them on. The lack of controlled trials and multiple variations of the procedure make it difficult to assess the true efficacy of the operation, but it has been shown to relieve angina subjectively and revascularize many patients objectively. The advent of direct coronary revascularization has had a dramatic effect in our ability to treat coronary artery disease, and its clear rationale overshadow the original murky concept of the IMA implant procedure. However, with the growing population of patients who are not amenable to conventional revascularization strategies due to unreconstructable coronary disease or due to failures following repeated direct coronary revascularizations, TMR is being explored as an alternative therapy. The advent of the TMR approach is re-kindling interest in the Vineberg operation, particularly on the underlying anatomical and physiological concepts. The unique historical contribution of Dr. Vineberg is being recognized, and this would, one suspects, greatly satisfy this courageous and persevering pioneer.

References

1. Shrager JB. The Vineberg Procedure: The immediate forerunner of coronary bypass grafting. Ann Thorac Surg 1994;57:1354-64.
2. Vineberg AM. Development of an anastomosis between the coronary vessels and a transplanted internal mammary artery. Can Med Assoc J 1946;55:117-119.
3. Vineberg AM, Miller G. Internal mammary coronary anastomosis in the surgical treatment of coronary artery insufficiency. Can Med Assoc J 1951;64:204-10.
4. Vineberg AM. Myocardial Revascularization by Arterial/Ventricular Implants. Massachusetts, John Wright/PSG Inc, 1982.
5. Vineberg A, Miller D. An experimental study of the physiological role of an anastomosis between the left coronary circulation and the left internal mammary artery implanted in the left ventricular myocardium. Surg Forum 1951;1:294-299.
6. Vineberg A, Miller D. Functional evaluation of an internal mammary artery coronary artery anastomosis. Am Heart J 1953;45:873-888.
7. Benscome SA, Vineberg A. Histological studies of the internal mammary artery after implantation into the myocardium. Am Heart J 1953;45:571-575.
8. Vineberg AM, Munro DD, Cohen H, Buller W. Four years' clinical experience with internal mammary artery implantation in the treatment of human coronary insufficiency including additional experimental studies. J Thorac Surg 1955;29:1-32.
9. Reis RL, Enright LP, Staroscik RN, Hannah H. The effects of internal mammary artery implantation on cardiac function and survival following acute coronary occlusion. Ann Surg 1970;171:9-16.
10. Vineberg AM, Lwin MM. Revascularization of both cardiac ventricles by right ventricular implants. Can Med Assoc J 1972;106:763-769.
11. Gorlin R, Taylor WJ. Selective revascularization of the myocardium by internal-mammary artery implant. N Engl J Med 1966;275:283-290.
12. Vineberg A, Deliyannis T, Pablo G. Myocardial nutrition after the Ivalon sponge operation. The return of a 400 million year old system. Can Med Assoc J 1959;80:949-958
13. Wearn JT, Mettier SR, Klumpp TG, Zschiesche LJ. The nature of the vascular communications between the coronary arteries and the chambers of the heart. Am Heart J 1933;9:143-164.
14. Vineberg A, Becerra A, Chari RS. The influence of the Vineberg sponge operation upon the hydrostatics of the myocardial circulation in health and disease. Evidence of luminal ventricular circulation in the beating heart. Can Med Assoc J 1961;85:1075-1090.
15. Vineberg A, Pifarre R, Mercier C. An operation designed to promote the growth of new coronary arteries using a detached omental graft: a preliminary report. Can Med Assoc J 1962;86:1116-1118.
16. Vineberg, A, Shanks J, Pifarre R et al. Myocardial revascularization by omental graft without pedicle: experimental background and report on 25 cases followed 6 to 16 months. J Thorac Cardiovasc Surg 1965;49:103-129.

17. Vineberg AM, Syed AK. The continuity of right and left ventricular myocardial sinusoidal spaces and its relation to right ventricular implants. Can Med Assoc J 1971;102:823-828.
18. Vineberg AM. Technical consideration for the combined operation of left internal mammary artery or right and left internal mammary artery implantation with picardiectomy and free omental graft. J Thorac Cardiovasc Surg 1967;53:837-847.
19. Buller WK, Vineberg A. A study of the amount of oxygen delivered to the myocardium through the implanted mammary artery. Surg Forum 1955;5:78-84.
20. Vineberg A, Kato Y, Pirozinsky WJ. Experimental revascularization of the entire heart. Am Heart J 1966;72:79-93.
21. Chiu CJ, Scott HJ. The Nature of Early Run-off in Myocardial Arterial Implants. J Thorac Cardiovasc Surg 1973;65:768-777.
22. Carlson RG, Edlich RF, Lande AJ, Bonnabeau RG, Gans H, Lillehei CW. A new concept for the rationale of the Vineberg operation for myocardial revascularization. Surgery 1969;65:141-147.
23. Baird RJ, Goldbach MM, De La Rocha A. The current status of the internal mammary artery implant operation. Vasc Surg 1975;9:647-651.
24. Vineberg A, Niloff PH. The value of surgical treatment of coronary artery occlusion by implantation of the internal mammary artery into the ventricular myocardium. Surg Gynecol Obstet 1950;91:551-561.
25. Vineberg A. Coronary vascular anastomoses by internal mammary artery implant. Can Med Assoc J 1958;78:871-879
26. Vineberg A. Evidence that revascularization by ventricular-internal mammary artery implants increases longevity. J Thorac Cardiovasc Surg 1975;70(3):381-397.
27. Bhayana JN, Gage AA, Takaro T. Long-term results of internal mammary artery implantation for coronary artery disease: A controlled trial. Ann Thor Surg 1980; 29:234-242.
28. Favaloro RG, Effler DB, Groves LK, Sones FM, Fergusson DJG. Myocardial revascularization by internal mammary artery implant procedures. J Thorac Cardiovasc Surg 1967;54:359-370.
29. Favaloro RG, Effler DB, Groves LK, Fergusson DJG, Lozada JS. Double internal mammary artery myocardial implantation: Clinical evaluation of results in 150 patients. Circulation 1968;37:549-555.
30. Sethi GK, Scott SM, Takaro T. Myocardial revascularization by internal thoracic arterial implants: Longterm follow-up. Chest 1973;64(2):235-240.
31. Gregori F, Toriano N, Oliveira SA, Carvalho RG, Galiano N, Macruz R, Verginelli G, Bittencourt D, Pileggi F, Zerbini EJ. Long-term results of mammary artery implants. J Cardiovasc Surg 1976;17:557-562.
32. Sones FM, Shirely EK. Cinecoronary arteriography. Mod Concepts Cardiovasc Dis 1962;31:735.
33. Vineberg A. Internal mammary artery implant in the treatment of angina pectoris- a three year follow-up. Can Med Assoc J 1954;70:367-378.
34. Vineberg A, Buller W. Technical factors which favour mammary coronary anastomoses with report of 45 cases of human coronary artery disease thus treated.

J Thorac Cardiovasc Surg 1955;30:411-435.

35. Kay EB, Demaney M, Tambe A, McLaughlin EE, Suzuki A. Internal mammary artery revascularization: Fact or fantasy. Chest 1973;64(2):227-233.

36. Ochsner JL, Moseley PW, Mills NL, Bower PJ. Long-term follow-up of internal mammary artery myocardial implantation. Ann Thor Surg 1977; 23(2);118-121.

37. Dart CH, Scott S, Fish R, et al. Direct blood flow studies of clinical internal thoracic (mammary) arterial implants. Circulation 1970;41&42 (suppl II):II-64.

38. Begg FR, Adatepe MH, Salvoza MI, et al. Myocardial scintigraphy: post-Vineberg study. J Thor Cardiovasc Surg. 1975;70:398.

39. Case RB, Nasser MG, Crampton RS. Biochemical aspects of early myocardial ischemia. Am J Cardiol 1969;24:766.

40. Fergusson DJ, Shirley EK, Sheldon WG, Effler DB, Sones FM. Left internal mammary artery implant-postoperative assessment. Suppl II Circulation 1968; 37&38:II-24-26

41. Sewell WH. The current status of surgery for coronary artery disease. Vasc Surg 1976;10:285.

42. Hayward RH, Korompai FL, Knight WL. Long-term follow-up of the Vineberg internal mammary artery implant procedure. Ann Thorac Surg 1991;51:1002-1003.

43. Topaz O, Pavlos S, Mackell JA, et al. The Vineberg procedure revisited: angiographic evaluation and coronary artery bypass surgery in a patient 21 years following bilateral internal mammary artery implantation. Cathet Cardiovasc Diagn 1992;25:218-222.

44. de Meester A, Leonard J, Chenu P, Marchandise P. Myocardial revascularization using Vineberg procedure; 23 year follow-up (French). Archives des Maladies du Coeur et des Vaisseaux 1994;87(9):1247-1248.

45. Salerno T. Cardioplegic arrest in patients with previous Vineberg implants. J Thorac Cardiovasc Surg 1979;78:769.

46. Nasu M, Takashi A, Hiroaki C, Shoumura T. Flow reserve capacity of left internal thoracic artery 23 years after Vineberg procedure. Ann Thor Surg 1996;61:1242-1244.

47. Tasdemir O, Kiziltepe U, Karagoz HY, Yamak B, Korkmaz S, Bayazit K. Long-term results of reconstructions of the left anterior descending coronary artery in diffuse atherosclerotic lesions. J Thorac Cardiovasc Surg 1996;112:745-754.

48. Mirhoseini M, Fisher JC, Cayton M. Myocardial revascularization by Laser: A Clinical report. Lasers in Surg Med 1983;3:241-245.

49. Hardy RI, Bove KE, James FW, Kaplan S, Goldman L. A histological study of laser-induced transmyocardial channels. Lasers Surg Med 1987;6:563-573.

50. Cooley DA, Frazier OH, Kadipasaoglu KA, Pehlivanoglu S, Shannon RL, Angelini P. Transmyocardial laser revascularization. Texas Heart Inst J 1994;21:220-24.

51. Kohmoto T, Fisher PE, Gu A, Zhu S-M, Yano OJ, Spotnitz HM, Smith CR, Burkhoff D. Does blood flow through Holmium:YAG transmyocardial laser channels? Ann Thor Surg 1996;61:861-868.

52. Tsang JC-C, Chiu RC-J. The Phantom of "Myocardial Sinusoids": A Historical Reappraisal. Ann Thorac Surg 1995;60:1831-1835.

53. Fleischer KJ, Goldschmidt-Clermont PJ, Fonger JD, Hutchins GM, Hruban RH, Baumgartner WA. One-month histologic response of transmyocardial laser channels with molecular intervention. Ann Thorac Surg 1996;62:1051-1058

54. Khouri RK, Brown DM, Hong S-P, Chung SH. Cytokine-induced internal mammary to coronary anastomosis. [Abstract]. Presented at the 1995 meeting of the Society of University Surgeons, Denver, CO, 1995:37.

55. Frazier OH, Cooley DA, Kadipasaoglu KA et al. Myocardial revascularization with laser: preliminary findings. Suppl II, Circulation 1995;92:58-65.

56. Cooley DA, Frazier OH, Kadipasaoglu KA, Lindenmeir MH, Pehlivanoglu S, Kolff JW, Wilansky S, Moore WH, Transmyocardial laser revascularization: clinical experience with twelve-month follow-up. J Thorac Cardiovasc Surg 111: 4, 791-7; discussion 797-9, Apr, 1996.

57. Vineberg A, Zamora B. A single artery implanted into the confluence of a tricoronary arteriolar zone in the left ventricular wall may revascularize the entire heart. Dis Chest 1969;56:501-518.

58. Trapp WG, Burton JD, Oforsagd P. Detailed anatomy of early Vineberg anastomosis. J Thorac Cardiovasc Surg 1969;57:451.

59. Baird RJ, Manktelow RT, Cohoon WJ, Williams WG, Spratt EH. Improved pressure gradients and flow rates in myocardial vascular implants. Ann Surg 1968;168:736-749.

3

TMR: IS IT STILL A PHYSIOLOGICAL IMPOSSIBILITY?

Roque Pifarré

Department of Thoracic & Cardiovascular Surgery, Loyola University Medical Center, Maywood, Illinois.

INTRODUCTION

The idea that we can tap the left ventricle to provide direct blood supply to the myocardium is very appealing. The fact that the left ventricle pumps oxygenated blood with each cardiac cycle, while the left ventricular myocardium is starving for oxygen when coronary artery disease is present, is not only puzzling but also frustrating. Therefore, many investigators have attempted to create functional channels that would supply oxygenated blood directly into the myocardial sinusoids and provide relief to the patients' angina.

In 1933, Wearn et al [1] described the existence of direct communications between the heart chambers and the myocardial sinusoids. He named them "arterioluminal" and "arteriosinusoidal" vessels. He suggested the possibility that, in the presence of coronary artery disease, the myocardium may be supplied with blood from the left ventricle through such vessels [2].

It is generally accepted that perfusion of the myocardium in the left ventricle takes place mostly in diastole. However, a systolic flow of a variable amount has been reported by Gregg et al [3]. They suggested that this blood stays in the epicardial arteries during systole and is readily available for quick myocardial entry with the onset of the next diastole.

Coronary artery flow is intimately related to the intramural pressure during the cardiac cycle. Quantification of the intramyocardial tissue pressure has been difficult, and different methods have been attempted. Pressure gradients from epicardium to endocardium have been reported by most investigators [3-5]. It has also been reported that tissue pressure in the deep layers of the left ventricular wall during systole exceeds the pressure recorded in the left ventricular cavity [4].

The importance of intramyocardial pressure to blood flow, during systole and diastole, cannot be overemphasized. The intraventricular pressure is lower than the intramyocardial pressure throughout systole and diastole. As a result, assuming this statement is correct, flow of blood from the left ventricle directly into the myocardium would be a physiological impossibility [6].

HISTORICAL PERSPECTIVE

Early Attempts At Direct Revascularization
The description by Wearn et al [1,2] of the "arterioluminal" and "arteriosinusoidal" vessels as direct communications between the heart chambers and the myocardial sinusoids was the concept that, later on, stimulated other investigators to attempt direct myocardial revascularization from the left ventricle.

Several investigators have attempted to apply Wearn's concept to revascularize the myocardium through artificially created channels with the left ventricle [7-14]. However, it has never been established whether blood flow, if any, occurs during systole or diastole. Several techniques were developed, including intramyocardial implantation of T tubes [8,9], boring [10] and needle acupuncture [11-14]. None of these techniques was successful. Thrombosis, scarring, or both, resulted in the occlusion of the created channels.

Intramyocardial Pressure
In 1968, we reported the recording of intramyocardial pressure during systole and diastole [15]. Pressures were recorded in an autogenous venous graft implanted in the left ventricular wall for the purpose of revascularizing the posterior myocardium, after producing ischemia with ameroid constrictors in the left anterior descending and the circumflex coronary arteries in the dog. This venous graft was anastomosed to the descending thoracic aorta and implanted with several branches open in the left ventricle. The end of the vein graft was left partially open as well (Figure 1). Anastomosis between the implanted venous graft and the coronary arteries were demonstrated radiographically (Figure 2). These pressure recordings,

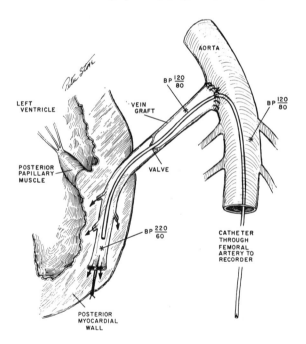

Figure 1. Schematic of a venous graft implanted in the posterior wall of the left ventricle. Pressures were measured in the aorta, in the portion of the vein graft outside the heart, and in the portion of the vein graft within the myocardium.

therefore, were believed to be a direct measurement of the intramyocardial pressure in the coronary system during the cardiac cycle. The pressure recorded intramurally in the graft must reflect pressures applied upon the intramural coronary arteries during the systolic myocardial contraction and during the diastolic relaxation (Figure 3).

In 1964, Kirk and Honig [4] concluded that peak systolic pressure in the inner half of the myocardium were greatly in excess of systolic intraventricular pressure.

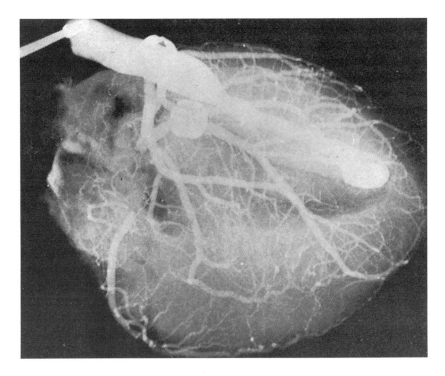

Figure 2. Radiograph of a heart made 3 months after implantation of an autogenous venous graft. Injection of the venous graft with Schlesinger mass filled the left coronary arteries.

Baird and colleagues [5,16,17] have studied extensively the intramyocardial pressure during the cardiac cycle. They reported that "the peak systolic intramyocardial pressure is higher near the inner wall of the ventricle than near the outer wall. Maximal peak systolic intramyocardial pressure may equal, but not exceed, the peak systolic pressure within the lumen of the left ventricle". They also reported that in patients with aortic stenosis, the intraventricular systolic pressure and the intramyocardial systolic pressure remains at normal or less than normal level. "Thus during almost all of systole, the deeper layers of the myocardial will be non-perfusable". In patients with coronary artery disease, "proximal coronary artery stenosis or occlusion will produce a diminution in distal coronary artery pressure during both systole and diastole. Such a lesion will not only reduce the total flow into the coronary artery, but will reduce the interval in the cardiac cycle

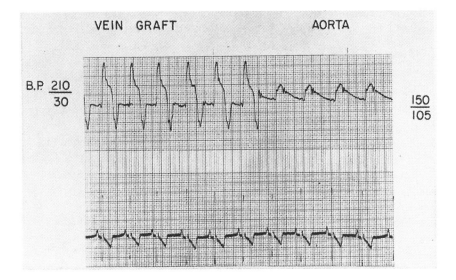

Figure 3. Pressure tracings recorded in the aorta and the intramyocardial venous graft.

during which the inner layers of the left ventricular myocardium can be perfused until, finally, only diastolic perfusion will be possible."

Experimentally, we demonstrated in 1968 [18], that when ischemia was induced with application of ameroid constrictors to the origin of the left anterior descending and circumflex coronary arteries in the dog, the implantation of a venous graft with branches and the distal end open, injection of the graft with Schlesinger mass revealed filling of the left circumflex artery at thirty days. After two months, injection of the graft filled the entire left coronary arteries (Figure 2). Although, at the beginning, the blood flows into the myocardial sinusoids, later it flows into the coronary arteries through collateral anastomoses.

The pressure measurements inside the tunnel showed that at the peak of systolic contraction, the pressure was 100 mm Hg higher than in the aorta and the left ventricle (Figure 1). During diastole, the pressure within the implanted vein was 20 mm Hg lower than in the aorta. These findings may be considered to provide a confirmation of the accepted physiologic principles of myocardial circulation. They seem to indicate that no flow of blood is possible, in the intramyocardial arteries, during the peak of systolic contraction. The lower pressure (that is, lower than in the aorta) during diastole may be a reflection of the myocardial perfusion during this phase of the cardiac cycle (Figure 3).

In 1969, we reported a study designed to evaluate the feasibility of direct myocardial revascularization from the left ventricle through artificially created channels [6]. The results obtained in this experiment were at variance with those reported by others [7,8,11,12]. The methods used by these authors varied considerably. Only one group used occlusion of the left circumflex artery as a challenging method [12]. However, the circumflex artery was ligated ten weeks later than the canalization was performed, and this group was compared with a control group that was submitted to acute occlusion of the same artery. In our hands, transmyocardial acupuncture and canalization by boring with Vim-Silverman needle did not reduce the high mortality rate or the size of the infarct as compared with those in the control group. Immediately, after the perforations were made, blood from the left ventricle came through the myocardial wall during systole. This bleeding was stopped by pressure or an epicardial suture. How much of this blood enters the myocardial sinusoids is not clear. However, even small amounts may have a beneficial effect in the ischemic myocardium in this acute phase. In the chronic survivors it was not possible to demonstrate, grossly or microscopically the patency of any of these perforations. The size of the infarct was similar to that of the control group.

The pressure measurements in an implanted venous graft in the posterior myocardium suggest that myocardial revascularization by transmyocardial acupuncture and canalization procedures is a physiologic impossibility. Simultaneous pressure recordings in the left ventricle, aorta, and the intramural segment of the implanted venous graft revealed that, during systole the pressure in the intramural segment of the implanted venous graft is greater than in the left ventricle and the aorta. During diastole it is lower than in the aorta but greater than in the ventricular lumen. These findings indicate that blood flow in the coronary arteries and perfusion of the myocardium take place during diastole. There is no possibility at any time during the cardiac cycle, systole or diastole, for blood flow from the ventricle to the myocardium [6].

MYOCARDIAL CHANNELS REVISITED

In 1981, Mirhoseini proposed creating transmyocardial channels with a laser apparatus [19]. High energy rather than mechanical means, were used to create channels [20]. The carbon dioxide laser used removes the tissue by vaporization. The authors evaluated the feasibility of using this laser to create channels in a beating heart. The laser energy could penetrate from the epicardium to the endocardium with, according to the authors, minimal damage to the surrounding tissue. Furthermore, the channel size could be controlled by the optical system.

The clinical use of the carbon dioxide laser was reported in 1988 by Mirhoseini et al [21]. They combined coronary bypass grafting with laser transmyocardial revascularization in twelve patients. They reported no mortality with a follow-up from three to thirty two months. Clinical improvement was noted in all patients. They report as a consistent finding the increased uptake of thallium isotope in the areas of revascularization by laser. According to them, follow-up left ventriculography demonstrated patent channels in six out of ten patients examined. They concluded that the clinical technique was safe, that the channels remained open and perfused the ischemic areas.

Yano and colleagues reported in 1993 the use of holmium:yttrium-aluminum garnet (YAG) laser to create nontransmural myocardial channels from the endocardial surface in the ischemic regions of the canine left ventricle [22]. In control dogs, the ischemic region was dyskinetic during the LAD ligation and reperfusion. In four of six laser-revascularized dogs, the regional preload recruitable stroke work remained positive in the ischemic region. They concluded that laser myocardial revascularization from the endocardial surface preserved regional myocardial function during acute ischemia.

Whittaker et al also experimented with the use of a holmium:YAG laser [23]. Transmural laser channels were made in dog hearts after ligating the left anterior descending artery. Transmural blood flow was measured before and after treatment using radiolabeled microspheres. They concluded that laser channels failed to increase blood flow to the ischemic area. There was no improvement in the regional myocardial function. Similarly, other studies have failed to find any benefit from the presence of laser channels [24,25].

Improved myocardial perfusion, relief of angina, and improved quality of life was reported by Mirhoseini et al in patients with diffuse coronary artery disease that were not candidates for aorto-coronary bypass [26]. These patients participated in an investigational treatment with a carbon dioxide laser to create transventricular channels. The follow up of this group of twenty patients ranged from two weeks to nine months.

Cooley et al described the histology of channels made by use of a carbon dioxide laser in a patient who died three months after treatment [27]. They reported vascular connections between the channels and the native myocardial vessels. They interpreted the long-term channel patency as indirect evidence of improved myocardial perfusion. Frazier et al reported their experience with sixteen cases treated with transmyocardial laser revascularization [28]. They concluded that this method of revascularization improved the clinical status and produced objective benefits at three months. Horvath et al described their experience with transmyocardial laser revascularization in 11 patients who were not candidates for PTCA or CABG and had persistent angina despite maximal medical therapy [29]. Although there were three postoperative deaths, they concluded that based on their results, transmyocardial laser revascularization may provide an alternative therapy for angina patients who cannot undergo PTCA or CABG.

More recently Whittaker et al obtained results that were consistent with the concept that channels were able to provide blood flow to the myocardium directly from the ventricular cavity; however, they did not document an increase in blood flow through the channels [30]. They concluded that the mechanism of protection is unknown. Kohmoto et al demonstrated that blood can penetrate into the myocardial wall directly through channels made with a pulsed holmium:YAG laser in the acute setting [31]. However, their results suggest that the flow is small, and based on the microsphere analysis, the gross appearance of the endocardium, and the histological appearance of the myocardium, the channels do not maintain connection with the left ventricular chamber after two weeks. The same group described similar histological finding in a patient who died four and a half weeks after transmyocardial laser revascularization, performed with a carbon dioxide laser [32]. The channels were occluded by granulation tissue, and there was no patent central passage in any channel examined. They concluded that since the channels created sealed off within two weeks, it would suggest that transmyocardial blood flow is not the mechanism that improves blood supply in the chronic clinical setting.

Cooley et al reported the use of an 800 W carbon dioxide laser used to drill 1 mm diameter channels into a beating heart after left thoracotomy, in twenty one consecutive patients [33]. Five patients died and thirteen were available for follow-up. Regional myocardial perfusion studies conducted using positron emission tomography indicated a significant change in relative subendocardial perfusion. The improvement in relative subendocardial perfusion is consistent with the clinical improvement observed in nine of eleven patients. The authors express doubts on how many of the laser-induced channels remain open for prolonged periods of time. They proposed the idea that the clinical and perfusional effects of the procedure may be due to other mechanisms; "the thermal, mechanical, or oxidative stresses associated with the insults may elicit adaptive responses and mediate angiogenesis in the laser-treated zones." Although, the precise contribution to blood flow is unknown, they believe that neovascularization occurs and may be important in the improved perfusion they reported. It should be pointed out that in the discussion of this paper that Mirhoseini, the originator of this method of revascularization, reported that angina subsides or disappears in most patients, but there is a rate of attrition two years after the operation. Although regional motion improves, the overall ejection fraction does not seem to change.

Horvath et al reported their experience with transmyocardial revascularization in twenty patients. Four deaths (20%) occurred within thirty days of the procedure [34]. One patient died six months after the procedure. The remaining fifteen did not require an increased dosage of medication from the preoperative levels. Compared with the preoperative baseline scans, there was a significant improvement in the areas of reversible ischemia. The authors report that subjectively the patients' symptoms improved immediately after the procedure and the improvement continued during the follow-up period. Objectively, the patients have shown improved perfusion in the treated areas. The perfusion improvement seems to be most apparent between three and six months. The authors admit that the exact mechanism that may improve perfusion and thereby provide relief of angina is unknown. They postulate that the TMLR channels and the energy delivered by the laser to the myocardium may stimulate angiogenesis. The process of angiogenesis would further improve perfusion by the formation of new collateral vessels.

As mentioned earlier, Burkhoff et al recently reported the autopsy findings obtained just over four weeks after operation [32]. The examination of the heart showed that the channels did not remain patent. Each channel consisted of fibrous scar and no channel showed any residual patent passage. The results in this patient indicate that TMLR channels did not remain patent. For this reason, the authors proposed that instead of blood flow from the ventricle to the myocardium, another mechanism has to be considered.

HAS ANYTHING CHANGED?

Myocardial Sinusoids
The concept of transmyocardial laser revascularization is based on the acceptance of Wearn and associates [1] description of the myocardial sinusoid, described as a run-off for coronary vessels that gradually loses its arterial character, resulting in a large vascular network. In 1946, Vineberg [35] applied this concept by implanting the internal mammary artery, with branches open, taking advantage of this large vascular network that would serve as an excellent run-off, allowing the formation of anastomoses with the coronary arteries that were partially or completely occluded proximally to the area of the implant. Direct communications between the implanted mammary artery and the coronary arteries were demonstrated angiographically by Effler et al [36]. The acceptance of the myocardial sinusoid concept combined with the recognition that the hearts of hayfish and lampreys lack coronary vessels, and are supplied directly by blood from the ventricular cavity, prompted Sen and associates to develop the idea of myocardial revascularization by transmyocardial acupuncture [11]. Taking it one step further, Mirhoseini and co-workers in 1982 attempted to create similar transmyocardial channels using a laser system [21].

However, with evolution, the direct nourishment of the myocardium by cavitary blood was replaced by the coronary arterial system. As the heart develops, the sinusoidal spaces become less important and partially obliterated, and the coronary arteries take on the main role of delivering oxygenated blood the myocardium. Chiu and Scott questioned the existence of the myocardial sinusoid [37]. They stated that "the irregular spaces seen in the histologic specimens of Wearn and others were probably distorted coronary veins, which may be distinguished by the presence of a rudimentary tunica intima, media, and adventitia". More recently, Tsang and Chiu reviewed the historical evolution as well as the validity of the concept of myocardial sinusoid [38]. They concluded by saying that "it is time that we cardiac surgeons give up the idea that the heart is a giant sponge!"

Blood Flow Through Channels
The key issues that have to be explained in relation to transmyocardial laser revascularization are the timing of the myocardial perfusion in relation to the cardiac cycle, and the pressure gradient between the left ventricular cavity and the ventricular myocardium. The proponents of TMLR assume that perfusion occurs in systole. It is well established that perfusion of the coronary arteries takes place in diastole. It is logical to assume that the same pressure gradients that regulate blood flow through the coronary vessels apply to the channels created by TMLR. According to several previously published investigations, the pressure in the intramyocardial coronary vessels is always higher than in the ventricle making it physiologically impossible to perfuse the myocardium from the ventricle [6,15,18]. We believe that the pressure measurements that were recorded in the implanted vein graft reflected the intramyocardial coronary artery vessels pressure, since we demonstrated communications between the vein graft and the coronary arteries. According to those recordings, the intraventricular pressure was never higher than the intramyocardial pressure, negating the possibility of blood flow to perfuse the myocardium through the TMLR created channels.

Channel Patency
The long-term channel patency is another controversial issue. Patency at the end of three months has been reported in a patient who died after TMLR [27]. The laser channels were assumed to be functional because they had endothelialized and contained red blood cells. In another reported case, whose autopsy was obtained four and a half weeks after TMLR performed with a carbon dioxide laser, the

channels were not patent [32]. The channels were occluded by granulation tissue. It will be necessary to clarify if the type of laser used makes a difference in the patency of the created channels. If it is proven that the created transmyocardial channels close in a short period of time, another mechanism will have to be found to explain the beneficial effects observed in some cases of transmyocardial revascularization. The results of the nuclear scanning study reported by Horvath et al suggest that the regional myocardial perfusion is improved in the areas treated by TMLR at six months, but not three months, after the procedure [34]. If the benefit was due to TMLR is should be immediate. Therefore, there is probably some other mechanism to explain the benefit of TMLR. The authors intimate that the energy delivered by the laser to the myocardium may stimulate angiogenesis, which would improve perfusion by collateral formation. Cooley et al reach the same conclusion that the clinical and perfusional effects of TMLR may be mediated through other mechanisms [33]. They refer to the works of Nakagawa [39] and Monte et al [40], that suggest that the thermal, mechanical, or oxidative stresses may elicit angiogenesis in the laser-treated zones.

SUMMARY

After review of the latest reports on TMLR, I believe it is safe to conclude that the clinical and physiological data presented by the authors support the idea that the possible benefit of TMLR results from augmenting regional collateral flow that follows angiogenesis in the laser-treated zones, and not from the passage of blood from the ventricular cavity to the myocardium, which continues to be a physiological impossibility clearly supported by the evolution of the species, as far as the development of the coronary circulation is concerned. The methods of channel-making may have changed, but the physiologic questions remain.

References

1. Wearn JT, Mettler SR, Klump TJ, Zschiesche LJ. The nature of the vascular communication between the coronary arteries and the chambers of the heart. Am Heart J 1933; 9:143-164.
2. Wearn JT. The role of the Thebesian vessels in the circulation of the heart. J Exp Med 1928; 47:293.
3. Gregg DE, Khouri EM, Rayford CR. Systemic and coronary energetics in the resting unanesthetized dog. Circ Res 1965;16:102-113.
4. Kirk ES, Honig CR. An experimental and theoretical analysis of myocardial tissue pressure. Am J Physiol 1964;207:361-7.
5. Baird RJ, Manktelow RT, Shah PA, Ameli FM. Intramyocardial pressure: A study of its regional variations and its relationship to intraventricular pressure. J Thorac Cardiovasc Surg 1970;59:810-25.
6. Pifarré R, Jasuja ML, Lynch RD, Neville WE: Myocardial revascularization by transmyocardial acupuncture. A physiologic impossibility. J Thorac Cardiovasc Surg 1969;58:424-31.
7. Goldman A, Greenstone SM, Preuss FS, Strauss SH, Chang ES. Experimental methods for producing a collateral circulation of the heart directly from the left ventricle. J Thorac Surg 1956;31:364-74.
8. Massimo C, Boffi J. Myocardial revascularization by a new method of carrying blood directly into the coronary circulation. J Thorac Surg 1957;34:257-264.
9. Pifarré R. An experimental evaluation of different procedures to induce ventricular=luminal myocardial circulation. Master of Science Thesis, McGill University, 1962.
10. Wakabayashi A, Little ST Jr, Connolly JE. Myocardial boring for the ischemic heart. Arch Surg 1967;95:743-752.
11. Sen PK, Udwadia TE, Kinare SG, Parulkar GB. Transmyocardial acupuncture. J Thorac Cardiovasc Surg 1965;50:181-189.
12. Khazei AH, Kime WP, Papadopoulos C, Cowley RA. Myocardial canalization. A new method of myocardial revascularization. Ann Thorac Surg 1968;6:163-171.
13. Sen PK, Doulatram J, Kinare SG, Udwadia TE, Parulkar GB. Further studies in multiple transmyocardial acupuncture as a method of myocardial revascularization. Surg 1968;64:861-870.
14. White M, Hershey JE. Multiple transmyocardial puncture revascularization in refractory ventricular fibrillation due to myocardial ischemia. Ann Thorac Surg 1968;6:557-563.
15. Pifarré R. Intramyocardial pressure during systole and diastole. Ann Surg 1968;168:871-875.
16. Baird RJ, Manktelow RT, Shah PA. The systolic pressure in the tunneled portion of a myocardial vascular implant. J Thorac Cardiovasc Surg 1969;57:714-720.
17. Baird RJ, Manktelow RT, Shah PA. Pressure in a vascular implant in the myocardium during systole. Circulation 1969;49:75. (Suppl I)

18. Pifarré R, Wilson SM, LaRossa DD, Hufnagel CA. Myocardial revascularization: Arterial and venous implants. J Thorac Cardiovasc Surg 1968; 55:309-319.
19. Mirhoseini M, Cayton MM. Revascularization of the heart by laser. J Microsurg 1981;2:253-60.
20. Mirhoseini M, Mucherheide M, Cayton MM. Transventricular revascularization by laser. Lasers Surg Med 1982;2:187-98.
21. Mirhoseini M, Shelgikar S, Cayton MM. New concepts in revascularization of the myocardium. Ann Thorac Surg 1988;45:415-420.
22. Yano OJ, Bielefeld MR, Jeevanadam V, Treat MR, Marboe CC, Spotnitz HM, Smith CR. Prevention of acute regional ischemia with endocardial laser channels. Ann Thorac Surg 1993;56:46-53.
23. Whittaker P, Kloner RA, Przyklenk K. Laser-mediated transmyocardial channels do not salvage acute ischemic myocardium. J Am Coll Cardiol 1993; 22:302-9.
24. Hardy RI, James FW, Millard RW, Kaplan S. Regional myocardial blood flow and cardiac mechanics in dogs with CO_2 laser-induced intramyocardial revascularization. Basic Res Cardiol 1990;85:179-97.
25. Landreneau R, Nawarawong W, Laughlin H, Ripperger J, Brown O, McDaniel W, McKown D, Curtis J. Direct CO_2 laser "revascularization" of the myocardium. Lasers Surg Med 1991;11:35-42.
26. Mirhoseini M, Cayton MM, Shelgikar S. Transmyocardial laser revascularization. J Am Coll Cardiol 1994;23 (suppl):416A. (abstract)
27. Cooley DA, Frazier OH, Kadipassaglu KA, Pehlivanoglu, Shannon RL, Angellini P. Transmyocardial laser revascularization: anatomic evidence of long-term channel patency. Texas Heart Inst J 1994;21:220-224.
28. Frazier OH, Cooley DA, Kadipasaoglu KA, Pehlivanglu S, Barasch E, Conger JL, Lindenmeir MH, Gould KL, Wilansky S, Moore WH. Transmyocardial laser revascularization: Initial clinical results. Circulation 1994;90 (suppl I):I-640. (abstract)
29. Horvath KA, Mannting F, Cohn LH. Improved myocardial perfusion and relief of angina after transmyocardial laser revascularization. Circulation 1994;90 (suppl I):I-640. (abstract)
30. Whittaker P, Rakusan K, Kloner RA. Transmural channels can protect ischemic tissue. Assessment of long-term myocardial response to laser-and needle-made channels. Circulation 1996;93:143-152.
31. Kohmoto T, Fisher PE, Gu A, Zhu SM, Yano OJ, Spotnitz HM, Smith CR, Burkhoff D. Does blood flow through holmium:YAG transmyocardial laser channels? Ann Thorac Surg 1996;61:861-8.
32. Burkhoff D, Fisher PE, Apfelbaum M, Kohmoto T, DeRosa CM, Smith CR. Histologic appearance of transmyocardial laser channels after 4 ½ weeks. Ann Thorac Surg 1996;61:1532-5.
33. Cooley DA, Frazier OH, Kadipasaoglu KA, Lindenmeir MH, Pehlivanoglu, Kolff JW, Wilansky S, Moore WH. Transmyocardial Laser Revascularization: Clinical Experience with Twelve Month Follow-up. J Thorac Cardiovasc Surg 1996;111:791-9.

34. Horvath KA, Mannting F, Cummings N, Shernan SK, Cohn LH. Transmyocardial Laser Revascularization: Operative techniques and Clinical Results at Two Years. J Thorac Cardiovasc Surg 1996;111:1047-53.

35. Vineberg AM. Development of an anastomosis between the coronary vessels and a transplanted internal mammary artery. Can Med Assoc J 1946;55:117-9.

36. Effler DB, Groves LK, Sones FM, Shirey EK. Increased myocardial perfusion of the internal mammary artery implantation: Vineberg's operation. Ann Surg 1963;158:526-34.

37. Chiu RC-J, Scott HJ. The nature of early run-off in myocardial arterial implants. J Thorac Cardiovasc Surg 1973;65:768-77.

38. Tsang JCC, Chiu RCJ. The phantom of "myocardial sinusoids": A historical reappraisal. Ann Thorac Surg 1995;60:1831-5.

39. Nakgawa K. Direct observation of laser-generated free radicals from a myocardium target site. Free Radical Biol Med 1992;12:241- 2.

40. Monte M, Davel LE, deLustig ES. Inhibition of lymphocyte-induced angiogenesis by free radical scavengers. Free Radical Biol Med 1994;17:259-66.

4

INCREASED PERFUSION VIA LASER-MEDIATED MYOCARDIAL CHANNELS?
Importance of Appropriate Models and Endpoints

Karin Przyklenk, Robert A. Kloner,
Peter Whittaker

Heart Institute, Good Samaritan Hospital and Department of Medicine, Section of Cardiology, University of Southern California, Los Angeles, California.

INTRODUCTION

Laser-mediated transmural myocardial revascularization (TMR) is being hailed as a promising new strategy for relieving myocardial ischemia in patients with diffuse coronary artery disease not amenable to bypass graft surgery or angioplasty. Indeed, anecdotal case reports and small clinical studies describing the merits of laser-mediated TMR are emerging in the literature [1-5], and the results of ongoing trials evaluating the efficacy of TMR are eagerly awaited. Surprisingly, however, the fundamental premise of the method -- ie. that laser-made channels serve as conduits for the transport of oxygen-rich blood from the left ventricular (LV) lumen to ischemic-but-viable myocardium, thereby restoring blood flow to the compromised tissue and resolving ischemic sequelae -- has not been rigorously confirmed in either the clinical setting or under the controlled conditions of the experimental laboratory.

Does laser-mediated TMR truly increase blood flow to ischemic myocardium and why, after fifteen years of investigation, does this seemingly simple question remain unresolved? Our objective in this Chapter is to apply the lessons learned from the discipline of myocardial ischemia/reperfusion to evaluate the current experimental evidence for and against increased perfusion via laser channels, with particular emphasis on the importance of the model chosen and endpoints measured when assessing the efficacy of laser-mediated TMR.

FIRST EVIDENCE: BENEFITS OF TMR IN ACUTELY ISCHEMIC CANINE MYOCARDIUM

In 1981, Mirhoseini and Cayton made the seminal observation that transmural channels made using a carbon dioxide laser dramatically improved survival in dogs subjected to acute coronary artery ligation [6]. Specifically, the authors found that 6/6 (100%) of control dogs succumbed to lethal ventricular fibrillation (VF) within 20 minutes of coronary occlusion while, in contrast, mortality was reduced to 0/6 (0%) in dogs receiving TMR before coronary ligation and 1/6 (17%) in the cohort "revascularized" at 5-10 minutes after the onset of occlusion. In addition, although the methods used to assess infarction were not specified, TMR was implied to salvage ischemic myocardium and limit infarct size: there was *"no evidence of infarct"* in dogs treated with TMR prior to occlusion, versus *"various amounts of gross infarct"* in both the controls and the TMR post-occlusion groups. The authors therefore concluded that *"channels created by the carbon dioxide laser effectively vascularize the myocardium so that it can meet the challenge of acute coronary artery occlusion"* [6]. This initial observation was supported by subsequent studies, again using the canine model, describing improved survival, attenuation of ST segment elevation, reduction of infarct size and preservation of contractile function in laser-treated hearts versus controls (Figure 1) [7-9]. Moreover, the results of Mirhoseini and Cayton have been credited in large part for providing the impetus for the clinical application of TMR.

RPRSW (mm Hg/sec/mm):

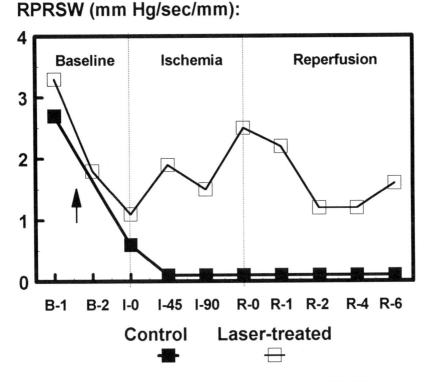

Figure 1. Average regional preload-recruitable stroke work (RPRSW: an index of contractile function) at B-1 (intact animals), B-2 (after laser application), I-0, I-45, I-90 (0,45 and 90 minutes after onset of myocardial ischemia) and R-0, R-1, R-2, R-4, R-6 (0-6 hours after coronary reperfusion) in the ischemic territory of control and laser-treated canine hearts. Arrow denotes time of laser treatment. Adapted with permission from reference [9].

THE CONFOUNDING VARIABLE:
VARIATION IN NATIVE COLLATERAL BLOOD FLOW

Does this impressive increase in survival, myocardial salvage and preservation of contractile function constitute proof of perfusion via the laser channels? It has long been appreciated that the incidence of lethal VF, and, in survivors, infarct size and recovery of contractile function are highly dependent upon both the severity of ischemia and the amount of myocardium rendered ischemic during coronary artery occlusion [10-14]. Thus, one interpretation of the TMR data is that laser-mediated channels did indeed supply blood flow to the jeopardized canine myocardium and thereby relieve ischemia.

There are, however, at least three other possible explanations. The first (and least explored) is that mechanical or thermal trauma caused by the laser may initiate an endogenous cellular protective response and render the myocardium resistant to a subsequent sustained coronary occlusion, analogous to the well-characterized phenomenon of "preconditioning" induced by one of more brief antecedent episodes of sublethal ischemia/reperfusion (reviewed in reference [15]). This potentially confounding issue might be of particular importance in TMR protocols involving laser irradiation applied immediately before a sustained occlusion of ≤ 90 minutes [8], as this is the time frame in which cardioprotection by ischemic preconditioning is manifest [15]. In this regard, Whittaker et al reported that **nontransmural** channels (ie. not perforating the subendocardial surface and thereby precluding the possibility of perfusion from blood in the LV cavity), made using a holmium:YAG laser, significantly reduced infarct size and attenuated the incidence of VF in rat hearts then subjected to a 1 hour sustained ischemic insult [16]. These data are consistent with the concept that acute thermal or mechanical injury induced by the laser may trigger a preconditioning-like effect.

The second potentially confounding factor is the extent of the occluded coronary artery bed, or "area at risk" of infarction. As might be expected, for a given severity and duration of ischemia, the total mass of necrotic myocardium and, in most models, the occurrence of life-threatening arrhythmias is greater in the setting of proximal coronary artery occlusion (involving, for example, 30% of the LV) than distal occlusion involving minimal amounts of the myocardium. For this reason, it is imperative in the dog and all other models to: (1) quantify the area at risk of infarction (ie. by injection of dyes or fluorescent particles); (2) confirm that the risk region is comparable in control versus laser-treated groups; and, for studies measuring infarct size (3) express the area of necrosis as a percentage of the area at risk [11,12,17].   Area at risk was not, however, rigorously measured or controlled for in the initial TMR studies [6-9].

The third and undoubtedly most crucial alternative explanation is based on a well-established hallmark of the canine model: that is, the inherent and extreme variability in native collateral blood flow in the dog heart. In ≈15-20% of dogs, coronary artery occlusion renders the myocardium profoundly ischemic, with blood flow to the ischemic territory uniformly reduced to ≈ 0 ml/min/g tissue.   In contrast, ≈5% of dogs have an extensive network of vessels connecting the left anterior descending and circumflex coronary beds, such that essentially normal blood flow is maintained via collateral channels despite total occlusion of a major coronary artery. This variability is illustrated in a recent retrospective analysis of 60 dogs compiled from 5 protocols in our laboratory, all involving 1 hour of coronary occlusion: 11 (18%) died of ischemia-induced VF, while 4 (7%) failed to develop ischemia [18]. The ≈75% of dogs that fall in the continuum between these two extremes are further characterized by a transmural gradient in collateral perfusion: ie. regional myocardial blood flow (expressed as mean ± SD) measured during occlusion in the remaining cohort of forty-five dogs was 0.06 ± 0.06 and 0.28 ± 0.24 ml/min/g tissue in the subendo- and subepicardial layers of the occluded territory, respectively [18]. Variability in the magnitude and transmural profile of collateral blood flow among animals is known to be a primary determinant of virtually all ischemia-related sequelae in the canine model. Not surprisingly, for example, for a given duration of coronary artery occlusion, there is a well-documented, significant inverse relationship between blood flow during occlusion and infarct size (Figure 2). For this reason, measurement of collateral blood flow -- and incorporation of collateral flow as a covariarte in statistical analyses -- is now regarded as *de rigeur* in canine ischemia/reperfusion protocols [11,12,18,19].

How does this variability in native collateral flow influence the interpretation of TMR results? Unfortunately, the reports of improved survival, myocardial salvage and enhanced recovery of LV function with TMR in the dog [6-9] were not accompanied by measurements of collateral perfusion. Thus, one cannot, with certainty, exclude the possibility that the superior outcomes in TMR-treated dogs may simply reflect differences in native collateral perfusion between control and laser-treated groups, rather than "revascularization" via the laser channels.

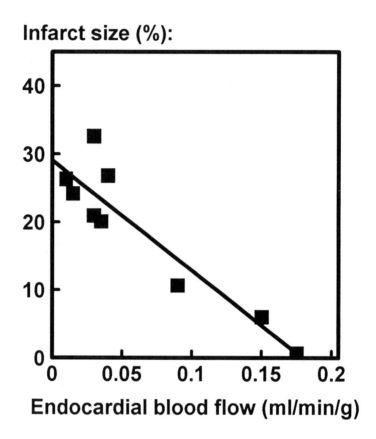

Figure 2. Infarct size (expressed as a percent of the area at risk) produced by one hour of coronary artery occlusion in the anesthetized canine model is dependent upon collateral blood flow to the ischemic subendocardium. Adapted with permission from reference [19].

ALTERNATIVE MODELS OF ACUTE ISCHEMIA

One method of avoiding the potentially confounding influence of variable native collateral blood flow inherent in the dog model would be to assess the acute effects of TMR in species known to have negligible and/or uniform collateral perfusion. Three models characterized in the ischemia/reperfusion literature as being rendered uniformly ischemic during acute coronary artery occlusion, with no transmural gradient in flow and little variation among animals, are the rat, the rabbit, and the pig, with mean transmural flows (± SD) averaging 12 ± 6% of normal nonischemic values, 0.03 ± 0.07 ml/min/g tissue (or ≈ 2% of nonischemic values) and 0.03-0.05 ml/min/g tissue (or 5 ± 3% of baseline flow measured before occlusion) in the three species, respectively [20-24].

In this regard, Goda et al found no benefit of channels made using the carbon dioxide laser in porcine hearts: there was no gross pathologic evidence of myocardial salvage with TMR and, in fact, the authors report a *"higher rate of early death"* in the laser-treated group [25]. In contrast, Horvath and colleagues described reduction of infarct size and improved recovery of contractile function with carbon dioxide laser treatment in sheep hearts, a model indicated by the authors to have no preformed collateral vessels [26]. Although the ovine model is not commonly used in ischemia/ reperfusion studies and is not well-characterized in terms of collateral blood flow, one study has reported that flow during coronary occlusion (mean ± SD) was 0.57 ± 0.24 ml/min/g tissue, or ≈44% of baseline flow measured before occlusion [27]. This implies that collateral flow in sheep is neither negligible nor uniform, and strongly suggests that the improved outcomes observed with TMR in both the canine and ovine models are plagued by the same potential uncertainties.

THE DIRECT APPROACH:
MEASUREMENT OF MYOCARDIAL BLOOD FLOW WITH TMR

A second and more direct approach to address the issue of flow via laser channels is to attempt to quantify changes in myocardial perfusion in response to TMR. For example, Whittaker et al randomly assigned dogs to receive holmium:YAG laser treatment or no intervention at thirty minutes after coronary artery ligation, and assessed regional myocardial blood flow in all dogs both before and after treatment. There were no differences in transmural blood flow between the two groups, and, in laser-treated dogs, perfusion to the ischemic myocardium before versus after "revascularization" was virtually identical (0.11 ± 0.04 versus 0.10 ± 0.03 ml/min/g tissue, respectively; Table 1) [28]. Similar conclusions were reached by Kohmoto and colleagues: in an elegant protocol designed to discern flow via laser channels from native collateral perfusion, the authors found that only 0.01 ml/min/g of flow could be attributed to laser "revascularization" [29].

Table 1.

Transmural myocardial blood flow (ml/min/g tissue) measured during left anterior descending coronary artery occlusion in anesthetized open-chest dogs

	Time post occlusion		
	25 min	**50 min**	**5½ h**
Control group:	0.12±0.03	0.11±0.03	0.15±0.04
Laser-treated group:	0.11±0.04 ↓	0.10±0.03	0.11±0.04

↓ transmural channels made at 30 minutes post occlusion using a holmium:yttrium-aluminum-garnet laser. No significant differences by 2-factor ANOVA (group and time) with repeated measures. Reprinted with permission from reference [28].

Both of these studies evaluated acute flow via channels made using the holmium:YAG laser and, despite the benefits seen by some authors with holmium:YAG and thulium-holmium-chromium:YAG treatment [8.9] , it has been argued that *"the holmium:YAG laser . . . is probably the worst laser for these procedures"* [30] because of the purportedly greater thermal injury associated with holmium:YAG versus carbon dioxide laser irradiation.   However, direct measurement of blood flow in canine hearts following carbon dioxide laser treatment also failed to yield evidence of augmented perfusion [31-33]. Even when left ventricular systolic pressure was elevated to > 200 mm Hg during brief and transient occlusion of both the left anterior descending and circumflex arteries, only a small increment in flow via the channels was noted [31].

A second criticism is that the method routinely used to measure myocardial perfusion in these TMR protocols and most ischemia/reperfusion studies -- that is, injection of 10-15 μm colored or radiolabeled microspheres which typically lodge in the microcirculation in proportion to the volume of flow received -- is not suitable for the accurate measurement of blood flow though laser channels [26,28]. In particular, the presence of radiolabeled microspheres trapped within a laser channel does not ensure that blood actually *circulates* from the left ventricular

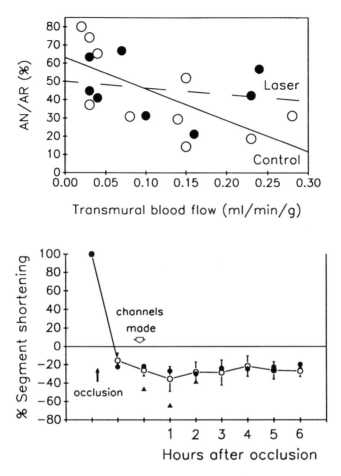

Figure 3: Top panel: Infarct size (area of necrosis [AN] expressed as a percent of the area at risk [AR]) plotted as a function of transmural collateral blood flow to the ischemic territory for control (open circles) and laser-treated dogs (solid circles) subjected to 6 hours of coronary artery occlusion. Laser treatment failed to reduce infarct size. **Bottom panel:** Regional segment shortening expressed as a percent of baseline preocclusion values and plotted as a function of time after occlusion. Open circles represent the mean value of 4 control dogs and the error bars show the SEM; solid symbols show data obtained from 2 laser-treated dogs. Laser treatment did not improve regional myocardial function. Reprinted with permission from reference [28].

lumen, through the channel, and into the surrounding tissue. Rather, the use of diffusible tracers (such as hydrogen clearance, or many of the tracers employed in positron emission tomography) may prove more useful in this regard [34]. However, in studies that employed the microsphere method and showed no change in regional myocardial blood flow with laser treatment, surrogate endpoints sensitive to the severity of ischemia, including infarct size, myocardial lactate concentrations, systolic contractile function, and depletion of high energy phosphate stores, also remained unchanged (Figure 3) [28,32]. Indeed, it is note-

Table 2. Comparison of laser revascularization studies in acutely ischemic myocardium.

Study	Laser Used	Model Used	Beneficial Effect	Blood Flow Measured
Mirhoseini & Cayton [6]	CO_2	Dog	Yes	No
Okada et al [7]	CO_2	Dog	Yes	No
Goda et al [25]	CO_2	Pig	No	No [†]
Jeevanandam et al [8]	THC:YAG	Dog	Yes	No
Hardy et al [31]	CO_2	Dog	No [¶]	Yes
Landrenau et al [32]	CO_2	Dog	No	Yes
Whittaker et al [28]	HO:YAG	Dog	No	Yes
Yano et al [9]	HO:YAG	Dog	Yes	No
Horvath et al [26]	CO_2	Sheep	Yes	No
Kohmoto et al [29]	HO:YAG	Dog	No	Yes
Kohmoto et al [33]	CO_2	Dog	No	Yes

† Flow measurements not required, as the pig is a model of low collateral flow
¶ small increase in flow via channels seen at high (>200 mm Hg) left ventricular pressure.
CO_2 = carbon dioxide; HO:YAG = holmium:yttrium-aluminum-garnet; THC:YAG = thulium-holmium-chromium:yttrium-aluminum-garnet. Adapted with permission from reference [28]

worthy that *improved outcome with laser-mediated TMR in the setting of acute coronary artery occlusion was only observed in those studies in which myocardial blood flow was not quantified* (Table 2), raising doubts as to the ability of laser channels to acutely "revascularize" ischemic myocardium.

RECONCILING THE PARADOX:
DOES TMR TRIGGER ANGIOGENESIS?

Despite the lack of proof of an *acute* increase in blood flow to ischemic myocardium through laser-made channels, improved perfusion (detected by thallium stress testing and positron emission tomography) has been described in some patients at *3-12 months post-operatively* [1-4,35] (Figure 4). In addition, autopsy reports from patients who died weeks to years following TMR have in some [1,2,4,36] (but not all [37]) instances revealed the presence of patent, endothelium-lined conduits with apparent vascular connections to the native coronary circulation. The obvious question is: how can these longer-term clinical observations be reconciled with the decidedly mixed results obtained during the initial hours following channel-making?

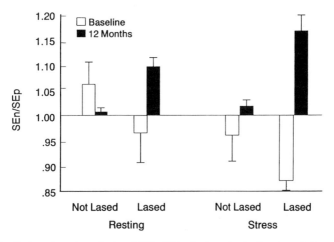

Figure 4: Subregional analysis of SEn/SEp (subendo-/subepicardial perfusion ratio) by positron emission tomography at rest (n=11 patients) and during dipyridamole stress (n=9 patients). Changes in SEn/SEp with respect to baseline was significantly different in lased segments compared with nonlased segments both at rest (p<0.0001) and under stress (p<0.01). Reprinted with permission from reference [35].

In an effort to resolve this paradox, Whittaker and colleagues proposed that laser-mediated TMR may stimulate the growth of new blood vessels which, over time, would connect the remaining lumen of the original laser channels with the existing microcirculation and eventually (ie. on the order of months, rather than minutes) provide a direct route for oxygen-rich blood from the LV cavity to reach the myocardium [38]. To test this concept, transmyocardial channels were made using a holmium:YAG laser in healthy, nonischemic rat hearts, a model characterized by uniformly low native collateral blood flow. *Two months later*, the rats were subjected to ninety minutes of coronary artery occlusion, the rationale being that myocardium receiving blood via new connections to the LV cavity should be protected, at least in part, from the sustained ischemic insult.

Indeed, there was a trend toward a reduction in infarct size in laser-treated hearts versus time-matched "sham-TMR" controls ($27 \pm 5\%$ versus $40 \pm 3\%$ of the myocardium at risk, respectively), with evidence of viable myocardium immediately adjacent to the laser channels [38]. Although this protection was not accompanied by an overall increase in capillary density, histologic analysis demonstrated the presence of 2-10 μm blood vessels "sprouting" from the lumen of several of the laser channels [38], analogous to the vascular connections alluded to in at least one clinical autopsy report [36]. Importantly, these vessels contained red blood cells which, in the absence of native collateral connections, presumably must have reached the ischemic territory via connections to the LV. It is interesting to note that even greater benefits were achieved in this same rat model when channels were made with either a needle [38] or an excimer laser [39] (Figure 5), raising the possibility that the reduced thermal and/or mechanical injury associated with these two methods versus the holmium:YAG laser may be an important determinant of the efficacy of laser-mediated TMR in both maintaining patency of the initial channel and triggering the progressive growth of new vessels from the original conduit [38,39].

In any case, the "delayed" protection seen two months after both laser and needle treatment is consistent with the concept that transmyocardial channels may provide a gradual (rather than immediate) supply of oxygenated blood from the LV cavity to the myocardium. It should be noted that, because these studies employed the rat model, interpretation of the data is not confounded by variations in native collateral blood flow. However, determination of the optimal strategies for channel-making, conclusive documentation of angiogenesis in response to TMR, and quantitation of blood flow via the new vessels all await further prospective study.

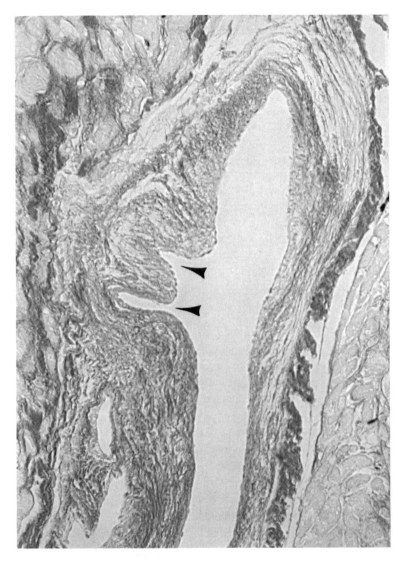

Figure 5. Micrograph of an open channel sixty-six days after it was made with an excimer laser. The width of the channel is approximately 65-86 μm. Two small vessels (10 μm in diameter) connect at right angles to the channel (arrowheads).

IN SEARCH OF THE ULTIMATE MODEL: "HIBERNATING" MYOCARDIUM

All of the experimental studies discussed in this Chapter have made a daunting demand of laser-mediated TMR -- that is, their objective was to determine whether laser channels can provide sufficient blood flow to salvage myocardium in the face of profound ischemia caused by abrupt and complete, mechanically-induced occlusion of an otherwise healthy coronary artery. TMR is not intended, however, as a clinical alternative to thrombolysis or angioplasty for the treatment of acute myocardial infarction, but rather as a strategy for providing oxygenated blood to so-called "hibernating myocardium" [40], a phenomenon characterized by chronic LV dysfunction at rest, presumably due to impaired myocardial perfusion through diseased and atherosclerotic coronary arteries, that can be partially or completely restored to normal by favorably altering the relationship between myocardial oxygen supply and demand. It is important to note that, in contrast to the rapid myocyte death initiated by abrupt coronary occlusion, the *hibernating myocardium remains viable* despite months-years of compromised perfusion, due in theory to an adaptive down-regulation and re-equilibration of metabolic activity and LV function to match the deficit in flow [40].

Since its first description in the clinical literature, investigators have sought to develop models of myocardial hibernation in the experimental laboratory by simple external application of a coronary artery stenosis. A state of steady low blood flow and accompanying metabolic down-regulation has, with some difficulty, been successfully maintained for a period of hours-days in both the canine and porcine models [41-44]. TMR has, to date, not been evaluated following acute subtotal coronary occlusion, but quantitative comparisons of myocardial perfusion with versus without laser channels would clearly be feasible in these models of so-called "short-term hibernation".

In contrast, efforts to maintain an experimentally-induced state of constant and prolonged low blood flow over the course of months, as described in patients, have failed. This is due in large part to the fact that prolonged sublethal ischemia is a potent and well-documented stimulus for angiogenesis (reviewed in detail in reference [45]), resulting in a progressive increase in tissue perfusion (rather than constant low blood flow) over time. Objective evaluation of TMR in models of long-term stenosis would therefore pose the intimidating challenge of definitively discerning flow via new vessels triggered by ischemia *per se* versus flow via new vessels initiated by channel-making.

A second confounding issue in both establishing valid long-term models of myocardial hibernation, and assessing TMR in these models, is that the definition and very existence of this phenomenon have been called into question. Specifically, there is both experimental and clinical evidence to suggest that the persistent LV dysfunction considered the hallmark of the hibernating myocardium may not be due, as first proposed, to constant and chronic low blood flow [40], but may be a consequence of chronic repeated episodes of transient and total coronary artery occlusion from which the heart never has time to fully recover [46,47]. Uncertainties in the etiology of chronic LV dysfunction do not, in themselves, preclude a future evaluation of TMR in this setting. However, as repeated brief ischemia is also recognized as a potent stimulator of angiogenesis [45], the same technical challenges inherent in models of long-term stenosis would apply to any efforts to conclusively document improved perfusion initiated by laser treatment in the setting of chronic repeated coronary occlusion. For these reasons, meaningful assessment of laser-mediated TMR in chronic experimental models of viable but hibernating myocardium is, at best, a distant goal.

LESSONS LEARNED AND FUTURE DIRECTIONS

In the fifteen years in which TMR has been evaluated in experimental models of acute myocardial ischemia, two important observations have emerged. First, as reviewed in Table 2, the weight of the current evidence strongly suggests that transumural channels made within minutes of total coronary artery occlusion using either a carbon dioxide or holmium:YAG laser fail, in themselves, to provide sufficient blood flow to "revascularize" and thereby salvage acutely ischemic myocardium. A second and equally important lesson is that conclusions regarding perfusion arrived at solely from measurements of arrhythmias, LV function, infarct size or any other surrogate indices of ischemia may at best be ambiguous or, at worst, misleading. This caveat is especially crucial for the evaluation of TMR in models (such as the dog) characterized by extreme variability in native collateral blood flow, in which there is simply no valid substitute for direct quatitative assessment of blood flow *per se*. However, the importance of direct measurement of myocardial perfusion in response to TMR extends beyond the setting of acute ischemia in the canine model: for example, if channel-making does in fact elicit a gradual improvement in blood flow by serving as a substrate for angiogenesis, conclusive proof of this hypothesis -- even in models, such as the rat, devoid of preformed collateral connections -- will ultimately be required. Despite the wealth of information available in the ischemia/reperfusion literature regarding measurement of myocardial blood flow, this issue is far from simple -- high-resolution methods capable of detecting *circulation* via laser-mediated channels must be applied. These experiments, if carefully designed using appropriate models and endpoints, will both resolve the lingering question of whether laser-mediated TMR truly augments blood flow to ischemic myocardium, and assist in the rational formulation of optimal strategies for future clinical applications of laser-mediated TMR.

References

1. Mirhoseini M, Shelgikar S, Cayton MM. New concepts in revascularization of the myocardium. Ann Thorac Surg 1988;45:415-420.
2. Mirhoseini M, Shelgikar S, Cayton MM. Transmyocardial laser revascularization: a review. J Clin Laser Surg Med 1993;11:15-19.
3. Horvath KA, Mannting F, Cohn LH. Improved myocardial perfusion and relief of angina after transmyocardial laser revascularization. Circulation 1994;90 (Suppl I):I-640. (abstract)
4. Frazier OH, Cooley DA, Kadipasaoglu KA, Pehlivanoglu S, Lindenmeir M, Barasch E, Conger JL, Wilansky S, Moore WH: Myocardial revascularization with laser: preliminary findings. Circulation 1995;92 (Suppl II):II-58-II-65.
5. Krabatsch T, Tambeur L, Lieback E, Hetzer R. Transmyocardial laser revascularization in the treatment of end-stage coronary artery disease. Ann Thorac Cardiovasc Surg 1998;4:64-71.
6. Mirhoseini M, Cayton MM. Revascularization of the heart by laser. J Microsurg 1981;2:253-261.
7. Okada M, Ikuta H, Shimizu K, Horii H, Nakamura K. Alternative method of myocardial revascularization by laser: experimental and clinical study. Kobe J Med Sci 1986;32:161-161.
8. Jeevanandam V, Auteri JS, Oz MC, Watkins J, Rose EA, Smith CR. Myocardial revascularization by laser-induced channels. Surg Forum 1990;41:225-227.
9. Yano OJ, Bielefeld MR, Jeevanandam V, Treat MR, Marboe CC, Spotnitz HM, Smith CR. Prevention of acute regional ischemia with endocardial laser channels. Ann Thorac Surg 1993;56:46-53.
10. Hale SL, Alker KJ, Lo HM, Ingwall JS, Kloner RA. Alterations in the distribution of high energy phosphates during ischemia in a canine model of reperfusion-induced ventricular fibrillation. Am Heart J 1985;110:590-594.
11. Reimer KA, Lowe JE, Rasmussen MM, Jennings RB. The "wavefront phenomenon" of myocardial ischemic cell death. II. Transmural progression of necrosis within the framework of ischemic bed size (myocardium at risk) and collateral flow. Lab Invest 1979;40:633-644.
12. Przyklenk K, Vivaldi MT, Schoen FJ, Arnold JMO, Kloner RA. Salvage of ischemic myocardium by reperfusion: importance of collateral blood flow and myocardial oxygen demand during occlusion. Cardiovasc Res 1986;20:403-414.
13. Bolli R, Zhu WX, Thornby JL. O'Neill PG, Roberts R. Time course and determinants of recovery of function after reversible ischemia in conscious dogs. Am J Physiol 1988;254: H102-H114,
14. Przyklenk K, Kloner RA. What factors predict recovery of contractile function in the canine model of the stunned myocardium? Am J Cardiol 1989;64:18F-26F.
15. Przyklenk K, Kloner RA, Yellon, DM. *Ischemic Preconditioning: The Concept of Endogenous Cardioprotection.* Boston: Kluwer Academic Publishers, 1994.
16. Whittaker P, Kloner RA. Myocardial preconditioning by laser irradiation. J Am

Coll Cardiol 1995;25:355A. (abstract)

17. Ytrehus K, Liu Y, Tsuchida A, Miura T, Liu GS, Yang XM, Herbert D, Cohen MV, Downey JM. Rat and rabbit heart infarction: effects of anesthesia, perfusate, risk zone and method of infarct sizing. Am J Physiol 1994;267:H2383-H2390.

18. Przyklenk K, Ovize M, Bauer B, Kloner RA. Gender does not influence acute infarction in dogs. Am Heart J 1995;129:1108-1113.

19. Przyklenk K, Sussman MA, Simkhovich BZ, Kloner RA. Does ischemic preconditioning trigger translocation of protein kinase C in the canine model? Circulation 1995;92:1546-1557.

20. Hale SL, Vivaldi MT, Kloner RA. Fluorescent microspheres: a new tool for visualization of ischemic myocardium in rats. Am J Physiol 1986;251:H863-H868.

21. Maxwell MP. Hearse DJ, Yellon DM. Species variation in the coronary collateral circulation during regional myocardial ischemia: a critical determinant of the rate of evolution and extent of myocardial infarction. Cardiovasc Res 1987;21:737-740.

22. Bankwala Z, Hale SL, Kloner RA. α-Adrenoreceptor stimulation with exogenous norepinephrine or release of endogenous catecholamines mimics ischemic preconditioning. Circulation 1994;90:1023-1028.

23. Savage RM, Guth B, White FC, Hagan AD, Bloor CM. Correlation of regional myocardial blood flow and function with myocardial infarct size during acute myocardial ischemia in the conscious pig. Circulation 1981;64:699-707.

24. Schaper W, Binz K, Sass S, Winkler B. Influence of collateral blood flow and of variations in MVO$_2$ on tissue ATP content in ischemic and infarcted myocardium. J Mol Cell Cardiol 1987;19:19-37.

25. Goda T, Wierzbicki Z, Gaston A, Leandri J, Vauron J, Loisance D. Myocardial revascularization by CO$_2$ laser. Eur Surg Res 1987;19:113-117.

26. Horvath KA, Smith WJ, Laurence RG, Schoen FJ, Appleyard RF, Cohn LH. Recovery and viability of an acute myocardial infarct after transmyocardial laser revascularization. J Am Coll Cardiol 1995;25:528-563.

27. Rezkalla S, Turi ZG, Keedy D, Precevski P, Kloner RA. Left main coronary angioplasty in a sheep model using a new left main autoperfusion balloon catheter. J Invasive Cardiol 1989;1:199-205.

28. Whittaker P, Kloner RA, Przyklenk K. Laser-mediated transmural myocardial channels do not salvage acutely ischemic myocardium. J Am Coll Cardiol 1993;22:302-309.

29. Kohmoto T, Fisher PE, Gu A, Zhu SM, Yano OJ, Spotnitz HM, Smith CR, Burkhoff D. Does blood flow through holmium:YAG transmyocardial laser channels? Ann Thorac Surg 1996;61:861-868.

30. Pfeiffer N. Will laser revascularization of the myocardium revolutionize treatment of heart disease? Two interpretations of the data. J Clin Laser Med Surg 1994;12:55-56.

31. Hardy RI, James FW, Millard RW, Kaplan S. Regional myocardial blood flow and cardiac mechanics in dog hearts with CO$_2$ laser-induced intramyocardial revascularization. Basic Res Cardiol 1990;85:179-197.

32. Landrenau R, Nawarawong W, Laughlin H, Ripperger J, Brown O, McDaniel W,

McKown D, Curtis J. Direct CO_2 laser "revascularization" of the myocardium. Lasers Surg Med 1991;11:35-42.

33. Kohmoto T, Fisher PE, Gu A, Zhu SM, Smith CR, Burkhoff D. Does blood flow through transmyocardial CO_2 laser channels? J Am Coll Cardiol 1996;27:13A. (abstract)

34. Fluck DS, Etherington PJE, O'Hare D, Winlove CP, Sheridan DJ. Myocardial tissue perfusion determined by particulate and diffusible tracers during ischemia: what is measured? Cardiovasc Res 1996;32:869-878.

35. Cooley DA, Frazier OH, Kadipasaoglu KA, Lindenmeir MH, Pehlivanoglu S, Kolff JW, Wilansky D, Moore WH. Transmyocardial laser revascularization: clinical experience with 12-month follow-up. J Thorac Cardiovasc Surg 1996;111:791-799.

36. Cooley DA, Frazier OH, Kadipasaoglu KA, Pehlivanoglu S, Shannon RL, Angelini P. Transmyocardial laser revascularization: anatomic evidence of long-term channel patency. Tex Heart Inst J 1994;21:220-224.

37. Burkhoff D, Fisher PE, Apfelbaum M, Kohmoto T, DeRosa CM, Smith CR. Histologic appearance of transmyocardial laser channels after 4½ weeks. Ann Thorac Surg 1996;61:1532-1535.

38. Whittaker P, Rakusan K, Kloner RA. Transmural channels can protect ischemic tissue: Assessment of long-term myocardial response to laser- and needle-made channels. Circulation 1996;93:143-152.

39. Whittaker P, Kloner RA. Excimer laser channels protect against myocardial ischemia. J Am Coll Cardiol 1996;27:13A (Abstract).

40. Rahimtoola S. The hibernating myocardium. Am Heart J 1989;117:211-221.

41. Fedele FA, Gewirtz H, Capone RJ, Sharaf B, Most AS. Metabolic response to prolonged reduction of myocardial blood flow distal to a severe coronary artery stenosis. Circulation 1988;78:729-735.

42. Przyklenk K, Bauer B, Kloner RA. Reperfusion of hibernating myocardium: contractile function, high energy phosphate content and myocyte injury after 3 hours of sublethal ischemia and 3 hours of reperfusion in the canine model. Am Heart J 1992;123:575-588.

43. Schulz R, Rose J, Martin C, Brodde OE, Heusch G. Development of short-term myocardial hibernation: its limitation by the severity of ischemia and inotropic stimulation. Circulation 1993;88:684-695.

44. Bolukoglu H, Liedtke AJ, Nellis SH, Eggleston AM, Subramanian R, Renstrom B. An animal model of chronic coronary stenosis resulting in hibernating myocardium. Am J Physiol 1992;263:H20-H29.

45. DeFily DV, Chilian WM. Methods for assessing coronary collateral growth: insights into mechanisms responsible for collateral development. In: *Collateral Circulation: Heart, Brain, Kidney, Limbs* (W Schaper & J Schaper, Editors). Boston: Kluwer Academic Publishers, 1993, p 29-40.

46. Vanoverschelde JLJ, Wijns W, Depré C, Essamre B, Heyndrickx GR, Borgers M, Bol A, Melin JA. Mechanisms of chronic regional postischemic dysfunction in humans: new insights from the study of noninfarcted collateral-dependent myocardium. Circulation 1993;87:1513-1523.

47. Shen YT, Vatner SF. Mechanism of impaired myocardial function during progressive coronary stenosis in conscious pigs: hibernation versus stunning? Circ Res 1995;76:479-488.

5

PHYSIOLOGY AND HISTOLOGY OF ACUTE MYOCARDIAL CHANNELS MADE WITH DIFFERENT LASERS

Takushi Kohmoto, Peter E. Fisher, Anguo Gu, Shu-ming Zhu, Carolyn DeRosa, Craig R. Smith, Daniel Burkhoff

Departments of Surgery, Pathology, and Medicine, Columbia University, New York.

INTRODUCTION

There is growing acceptance of the use of transmyocardial laser revascularization (TMLR) to treat patients with angina that is refractory to conventional therapies [1-3]. This acceptance is largely based upon the fact that ongoing clinical trials have consistently shown that TMLR provides a significant reduction in angina [1, 4-9]. Importantly, this rather dramatic effect on chest pain is not short-lived as might be expected with either a placebo effect or with the previously observed transient relief of angina seen after thoracotomy [10]. Furthermore, there is also evidence that over time, regional blood flow is improved in myocardium treated with TMLR

[5,6,9]. Despite these encouraging clinical results, there is still significant controversy over the mechanisms of both the relief of angina and improved blood flow.

In an effort to understand the acute effects of TMLR on regional myocardial perfusion, we have performed studies in isolated cross-perfused and intact canine hearts using two different types of lasers: a carbon dioxide laser and a holmium:YAG laser. As will be described in detail below, the isolated heart preparation offers the advantage of being able to separate transmyocardial blood flow from coronary blood flow to test directly whether and how much blood flows acutely through TMLR channels. In order to further investigate the subacute effects of TMLR, myocardial tissue was also examined two weeks after making the channels. This chapter summarizes our observations concerning the physiology and histology of TMLR channels made with these two types of laser [11-15].

ISOLATED HEART STUDIES

Isolated heart studies were performed to test specifically whether acute myocardial perfusion could be achieved through TMLR channels. Laser channels were created in hearts of mongrel dogs and then studied after being isolated and cross-perfused by blood circulating from a second support dog using methods that have been described previously [14]. In brief, the support dog was anesthetized (pentobarbital sodium 30 mg/kg administered intravenously), heparinized (5,000 U intravenous bolus), intubated, and mechanically ventilated. The femoral arteries and veins were cannulated and connected to a perfusion system which was used to supply oxygenated blood to isolated hearts. The heart donor dog was also anesthetized, anticoagulated, mechanically ventilated, and a left thoracotomy was performed. TMLR channels were then created over the antero-lateral region of the heart; that is, the region supplied by the distal left anterior descending (LAD) artery. A carbon dioxide laser (The Heart Laser, PLC Systems, Milford, MA) was used in five dogs and a holmium:YAG laser (CardioGenesis Corporation, Sunnyvale, CA) was used in an additional five. With the carbon dioxide laser, each channel was made with a 40 J pulse, which is the average energy used in the ongoing clinical trials. The holmium:YAG laser delivers 2 J per pulse through a fiber optic cable (CardioGenesis Corporation, Sunnyvale, CA). Approximately 12-18 pulses are required to make each channel using the holmium:YAG laser system. Thus, the total energy delivered was 24-36 J per channel. In all cases, channels were made with a density of approximately one per square centimeter and an average of 12 (range 11-13) channels were made in each heart.

After lasing, and with the heart still in situ, all visible epicardial collaterals were ligated with 5-0 suture to minimize collateral flow to the distal LAD territory. Thirty minutes after creating the channels, a medial sternotomy was performed, the heart was excised, and connected to the perfusion apparatus for cross-perfusion.

In order to control the left ventricular volume and pressure of the isolated hearts, a large bore cannula (28F) connected to a reservoir was introduced into the left ventricular chamber via the left atrial appendage. After completing this preparation of the heart, the LAD was ligated and the heart was allowed to stabilize for an additional twenty minutes prior to starting the protocol.

In this isolated heart preparation, the aortic valve was kept shut either by keeping the aortic pressure greater than the ventricular pressure (holmium:YAG studies) or by suturing the aortic valve cusps (carbon dioxide studies). Since the aortic valve was closed, there was no possibility for the coronary and ventricular blood to mix. Accordingly, substances put into the coronary blood appear in the myocardium solely as a result of coronary flow, and substances put into blood within the ventricular chamber appear in the myocardium solely as a result of transmyocardial flow. In the studies described here, we put microspheres of different colors into the coronary and ventricular blood.

Colored microspheres (15 μm diameter; approximately 3×10^6 microspheres/ mL in a saline suspension with 0.01% Tween 80 and thimerosal; Dye-Trak, Triton Technology, Inc., San Diego, CA) were used to estimate regional coronary artery flow and to detect blood flow through the channels. In each experiment, injections of four different colored microspheres (white, yellow, red, and blue) were used to measure regional blood flows under four different conditions. Regional blood flow from the normal coronary vasculature was determined at the start of the protocol by injecting 0.2 mL of the first set of colored microspheres into the coronary arterial perfusion line. Next, microspheres were injected into blood placed within the LV chamber under to different loading conditions that were applied in a random order among the hearts. One condition was a low loading condition in which peak LV pressure generation was approximately 20 mm Hg, and the other was a high loading condition in which peak LV pressure generation ranged between 80 and 100 mm Hg. For each condition, a total of 2.5 mL of the mixed microspheres were injected (a total dose of 7.5×106 spheres) for ten minutes, after which the LV chamber was emptied and filled with fresh blood. The two loading conditions were studied because if appreciable perfusion can be achieved through TMLR channels then, as suggested by some investigators [1,2], perfusion should be greater at the high load as compared to the low load. A 1 mL sample of LV blood was obtained during the period of percolation (for determination of blood microsphere concentration). After performing the intraventricular injections at both loading conditions, a final set of microspheres (0.2 mL) was injected into the coronary artery to measure the collateral blood flow. This was done to test whether there was any change in collateral flow into the LAD territory over the duration of the experiment.

At the end of the experiment, the heart was removed from the perfusion system and cut into small samples (approximately 1 g in mass) from the laser-treated region of the LAD territory and from the perfusion territory of the left circumflex artery. Retrieval and quantitative analysis of the microspheres were performed as described previously [14,16].

Assessment of Acute Blood Flow Using a Physiologic End-point
The goal of the protocol described above was to obtain direct evidence of myocardial perfusion through TMLR channels. In order to obtain corroborating evidence of blood flow through TMLR channels using a physiologic end-point, we examined whether acute TMLR channels could protect against an acute LAD ligation. This protocol was performed only with the carbon dioxide laser because a similar study had already been donee with a holmium:YAG laser [17]. Under general anesthesia, a left thoracotomy was performed and the pericardium was opened. Using the carbon dioxide laser with a pulse energy of 40 J, TMLR channels were made at a density of one per square centimeter (an average of 10 channels per heart) in the territory supplied by the LAD after the takeoff of the first diagonal branch. The LAD and all of the visible epicardial collaterals to this territory were ligated. The thoracotomy was closed and the animal recovered from anesthesia. Twenty-four hours after occlusion, the animals were euthanized and the heart excised. The myocardium was sliced into three layers; the subepicardial outer third, the subendocardial inner third, and the middle third. The middle layers were incubated in a solution of triphenyltetrazolium chloride, which specifically allows differentiation of viable from non-viable myocardium. The subepicardial and subendocardial layers were fixed overnight by immersion in 10% neutral buffered formalin before dehydration and paraffin embedding. Histologic sections were stained with hematoxylin and eosin and with trichrome and examined microscopically.

Histologic Appearance of TMLR Channels Two Weeks After Creation in Normal and Infarcting Myocardium

To evaluate the long-term morphology of TMLR channels, a total of ten dogs were treated with the carbon dioxide laser and an additional four dogs with the holmium:YAG laser, using surgical and laser procedures identical to those described above for the twenty-four hour study. An average of seventeen channels (approximately one per square centimeter) were made over the distal LAD distribution as described above. In half of the animals, the LAD was ligated (with 3-0 silk) just distal to the first diagonal branch. The chest was closed and the dogs allowed to recover. Two weeks after operation, the animals were euthanized (all of the animals survived to the end of the protocol), and the hearts excised as described above.

ACUTE PERFUSION RESULTS

The microscopic appearance of typical acute channels made with the carbon dioxide laser and with the holmium:YAG laser in normal canine myocardium are illustrated in Figure 1 (with hematoxylin and eosin staining). The channel lumens were similar with both lasers. Surrounding each channel was a zone of thermal necrosis (demarcated by the arrows in Figure 1) which, as expected was slightly greater with the holmium:YAG laser.

Absorbance spectra of samples retrieved from myocardium in the non-lased circumflex region were examined from every dog studied to determine whether there was any non-specific microsphere uptake into the myocardium. These spectra never revealed any microsphere density greater than the noise level inherent to the colored microsphere technique [16]. A typical example is shown in Figure 2A. A spectrum obtained from myocardium of the LAD territory which was lased with the holmium:YAG laser is shown in Figure 2B. In this example, white and red spheres were injected into the coronary arteries, while yellow and blue spheres were injected directly into the ventricular chamber. Since there are peaks corresponding to yellow and blue, these findings indicate that transmyocardial and native coronary blood flows were separated and that microspheres can reach the myocardium by passing directly through the laser channels. Spectra obtained from myocardium lased with the carbon dioxide laser system were generally similar in

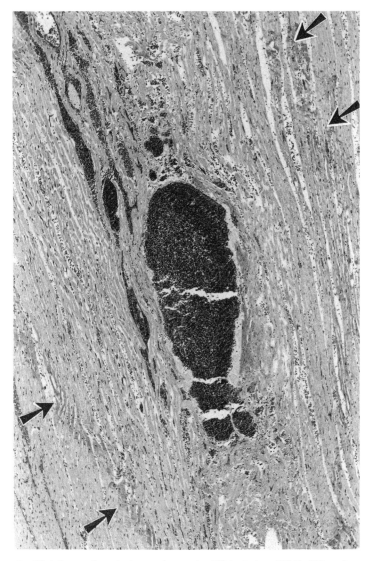

Figure 1. Histology of acute laser channels; (A) holmium:YAG, (B) carbon dioxide. Sections stained with hematoxylin and eosin. Both channels contain a central tissue-ablated core, marginal lacunar changes immediately surrounding the channels, and a circumferential zone of thermal and thermoacoustic damage (demarcated by the arrows).

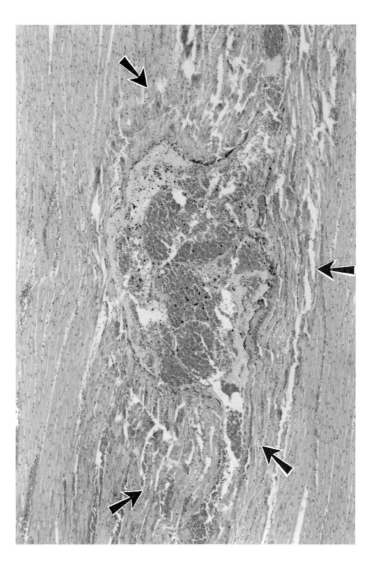

Figure 1B. Channel made with a carbon dioxide laser.

appearance, though on a quantitative basis the peaks corresponding to transmyocardial flow were lower.

In order to provide a quantitative estimate of transmyocardial flow, microsphere numbers were determined from the spectra and these were then converted into flows (details of these quantitative methods have been provided previously [14]). The results obtained for both holmium:YAG and carbon dioxide studies are summarized in Table 1. Note that we found no difference between the high and low pressure loading conditions for either laser and so the results are not distinguishable in the table.

Table 1. Myocardial perfusion from different sources into the distal LAD territory after the creation of laser channels and after ligation of the LAD and epicardial collateral vessels.

Laser	Coronary blood flow (mL/min)	Transmyocardial flow (mL/min)
holmium:YAG	0.26±0.17	0.0010±0.0008*
carbon dioxide	0.11±0.07	0.0018±0.0014

* significantly different than transmyocardial flow determined in the non-lased circumflex region.

The LAD and epicardial collateral artery ligations resulted in myocardial flows which were approximately 15% of normal, indicating that we were successful in markedly decreasing coronary flow to the laser treated regions. While the microsphere numbers resulting from transmyocardial flow were increased in the laser-treated regions, particularly after treatment with the holmium:YAG laser, the amount of myocardial perfusion achieved through the channels was exceedingly small. Although this increase was statistically significant for the holmium:YAG laser, it was of no physiologic significance.

Myocardial Viability at Twenty-four Hours After Treatment
Myocardial tissue was examined from four dogs which underwent LAD and epicardial collateral ligation and subsequent treatment with the carbon dioxide laser. The treated areas were stained with TTC and samples were also obtained for

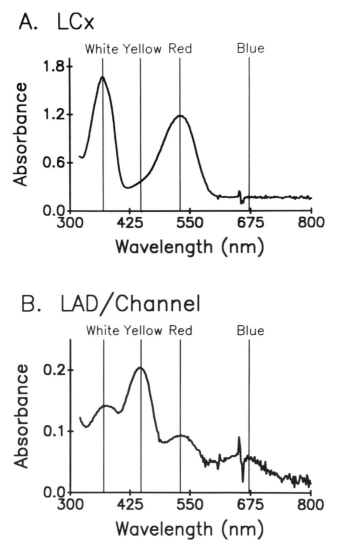

Figure 2. Typical spectra from an acute (holmium:YAG) isolated heart study in which white and red spheres were injected into the coronaries and yellow and blue spheres were injected into the LV cavity. The spectrum in panel A is from the non-lased, normally perfused circumflex territory. The spectrum in panel B is from the LAD territory which was rendered ischemic and in which channels were created with a holmium:YAG laser. See text for further details.

routine histologic examination. The channels were all patent and maintained a connection with the left ventricular chamber, as was evident upon gross inspection of the endocardial surface. TTC staining of tissue surrounding the channels in the ischemic zone was completely white (viable muscle stains red), indicating a lack of any viable myocardium around channels in this region. This finding was confirmed by examination of the histologic sections stained with trichrome, which failed to show any viable myocytes around the channels. These observations suggest that blood flow, if any, through acute TMLR channels was not physiologically significant.

Long-term Appearance of TMLR Channels
At two weeks after treatment, there was no significant difference between the microscopic appearance of myocardium treated with the carbon dioxide laser and that treated with the holmium:YAG laser. Epicardial scars were identified at the original laser entry sites in hearts of animals that were lased but in which the LAD was not ligated. In addition, most of the channels were identified by shallow epicardial stitches. Upon opening the LV chamber, small elliptical endocardial scars could be identified which likely represent the original entry point of the laser channel into the LV cavity. There were no widely open channel entry points which appeared macroscopically to represent the location of the channels on the endocardial surface. Typically, the original channel region was invaded with granulation tissue containing lacunar spaces filled with fibrin. These spaces were typically endothelialized (confirmed by staining with antibodies for Factor VIII) and also contained red blood cells. The larger of these lacunar spaces typically ranged in size between 50 and 75 μm in diameter. These regions also typically contained many capillaries and small arteries in their centers. Furthermore, and importantly, there was also a significant increase in the number of small arteries (that is, arteries containing one or more layers of smooth muscle cells) in normal myocardium surrounding the channel remnants [18].

In tissue examined two weeks after lasing with simultaneous LAD ligation, many channels were obscured by the massive healing response incited by the occlusion-related infarction. For this reason, no definitive channels were identified within the actively healing myocardium of these infarcted regions. Furthermore, as would be expected from the results obtained after only twenty-four hours, there was no viable myocardium identified around areas in which channels were identified.

DISCUSSION

The goal of the studies described in this chapter was to prove that blood does flow through TMLR channels. Such a finding would support the prevailing theory of TMLR. A positive result (that is, confirmation of that hypothesis) using the present techniques would undoubtedly have been easily accepted by the TMLR research community. However, the results did not confirm the hypothesis. In view of the importance of TMLR as a current research topic, a negative finding, should be made available for all investigators to consider. We used multiple experimental approaches in recognition of the possibility that any one of the approaches may have limitations (as indeed does any experimental study in animals); the results from all of the approaches were unambiguous and internally consistent. These findings are important and, we contend, do pertain to the clinical situation (discussed below). It is important to emphasize that the negative results of this study do not challenge the encouraging clinical results obtained with the technique, nor do they in any way jeopardize the potential development and thorough evaluation of this technology in the clinical setting.

Importantly, there was no physiologically significant difference noted between the characteristics of the holmium:YAG and carbon dioxide lasers, with the exception of the amount of thermal damage noted in the acute TMLR channels (the damage was greater with the holmium:YAG laser). The clinical significance of the latter finding would appear to be negligible, since when viewed two weeks later, the channel remnants associated with the two lasers were indistinguishable.

The results of the present study are consistent with those of some previous studies which concluded that there was no significant blood flow through acute TMLR channels [14,17,19,20]. In one study, TMLR channels made with a holmium:YAG laser failed to preserve myocardial viability around the channels after a six hour LAD ligation [17]. Two other studies, which employed different types of carbon dioxide laser, also failed to demonstrate any acute increase in myocardial perfusion due to TMLR channels [19,20]. Finally, one group if investigators reasoned from studies of the physiology of blood flow within the myocardium that blood flow through transmyocardial channels was a physiologic impossibility [21]. Although in the particular case considered, the channels were made with needles, the same physiologic arguments would apply to channels made by any means.

In contrast, results of several studies suggest that the presence of TMLR channels confers a physiologic benefit, particularly in the chronic setting [22-24]. Most notable of these studies was a recent investigation by Whittaker et al in which transmyocardial channels made with needles and a holmium:YAG laser in rat hearts were patent two months after their creation (although with a caliber significantly reduced from the acute setting) [25]. Two months after creation of the channels, they ligated the left coronary artery to make the channel-treated region ischemic and injected particulate pigment into the femoral vein. Although the pigment was found in the channels, the density of pigment as appreciably lower than in the non-ischemic regions of the heart. This observation suggests that any blood flow through the patent channels was small. However, the presence of needle, but not laser, channels also conferred a benefit in that the infarct size observed in the face of an acute left coronary artery occlusion was reduced versus that found in control (untreated) hearts. This finding suggests that blood flow through the channels was physiologically relevant.

The present studies examined flow potential and histology only in acute (within twenty-four hours) and subacute (up to two weeks) settings. While the clinical experience is related more to the setting of chronic ischemia and the long-term relief of angina, understanding gleaned from the current studies provides information which is potentially vital to the clinical understanding of the procedure in several respects. First, angina relief follows quickly after the surgery; patients typically leave the hospital with significantly reduced or even no angina [6,7]. Second, preliminary clinical experience reveals relatively high perioperative mortality and morbidity in patients with unstable angina. Third, this perioperative morbidity is mostly related to myocardial infarction. These and other factors render it imperative, at least as a first step, to understand the acute blood flow potential through TMLR channels. As discussed above, results of recent studies in rats suggest that over longer time periods (months rather than weeks), TMLR channels confer a statistically significant benefit in terms of myocardial protection in the face of subsequent coronary artery ligation [25] which is not apparent in the acute setting. These important findings suggest that the physiology of acute and chronic channels likely differ, a notion that needs to be investigated thoroughly.

As stated above, experimental studies, such as described here, address issues of mechanism of action and do not address issues of clinical effectiveness. Therefore, the negative findings of lack of physiologically significant acute channel blood flow and apparent morphologic change at two weeks do not in any way suggest a lack of clinical efficacy. Nevertheless, it is of significant importance that the mechanism of clinical benefit of TMLR be elucidated. Such information may be useful for devising means of identifying patients most likely to benefit from the procedure. Furthermore, questions related to optimizing laser parameters (for example, wavelength, pulse characteristics etc) will provide equal clinical benefit can be more effectively addressed once the mechanism of benefit is defined. To the degree that the present results pertain to the clinical setting, the results suggest that mechanisms other than blood flow through TMLR channels be considered in future studies.

Acknowledgment

These studies were supported by funds provided by CardioGenesis Corporation, Sunnyvale, CA and from the Departments of Surgery and Medicine of the Columbia Presbyterian Medial Center. DB was supported by a grant from the American Heart Association, New York City Affiliate and from the Whitaker Foundation.

94 Direct Myocardial Revascularization

References

1. Mirhoseini M, Shelgikar S, Cayton MM. New concepts in revascularization of the myocardium. Ann Thorac Surg 1988;45:415-420.
2. Mirhoseini M, Cayton MM, Shelgikar S, Fisher JC. Clinical report: laser myocardial revascularization. Lasers Surg Med 1986;6:459-461.
3. Cooley DA, Frazier OH, Kadipasaoglu KA, Pehlivanoglu S, Shannon RL, Angelini P. Transmyocardial laser revascularization: anatomic evidence of long-term channel patency. Tex Heart Inst J 1994;21:220-224.
4. Cooley DA, Frazier OH, Kadipasaoglu KA, Pehlivanoglu S, Barasch E, Conger JL, Lindenmeir MH, Gould KL, Wilansky S, Moore WH. Transmyocardial laser revascularization: initial clinical results. Circulation 1994;90 (suppl I):I-640. (abstract)
5. Horvath KA, Mannting F, Cohn LH. Improved myocardial perfusion and relief of angina after transmyocardial laser revascularization. Circulation 1994;90 (Suppl I) :I-640. (abstract)
6. Frazier OH, Cooley DA, Kadipasaoglu KA, Pehlivanoglu S, Lindenmeir M, Barasch E, Conger JL, Wilansky S, Moore WH. Myocardial revascularization with laser: preliminary findings. Circulation 1995;92 (Suppl II):II-58-II-65.
7. Cooley DA, Frazier OH, Kadipasaoglu KA, Lindenmeir MH, Pehlivanoglu S, Kolff JW, Wilansky S, Moore WH. Transmyocardial laser revascularization: clinical experience with twelve-month follow-up. J Thorac Cardiovasc Surg 1996;111:791-799.
8. Krabatsch T, Dörschel K, Tülsner J, Hempel B, Hofmeister J, Lieback E, Hetzer R. Transmyocardial laser revascularization - initial results in treating diffuse coronary disease. Lasermedizin 1995;11:192-198.
9. Horvath KA, Mannting F, Cummings N, Shernan SK, Cohn LH. Transmyocardial laser revascularization: operative techniques and clinical results at two years. J Thorac Cardiovasc Surg 1996:111:1047-1053.
10. Dimond EG, Kittle CF, Crockett JE. Comparison of internal mammary artery ligation and sham operation for angina pectoris. Am J Cardiol 1960:5:483-486.
11. Kohmoto T, Burkhoff D, Yano OJ, Fisher PE, Spotnitz HM, Smith CR. Demonstration of blood flow through transmyocardial laser channels. J Am Coll Cardiol 1995;25:7A. (abstract)
12. Burkhoff D, Fisher PE, Apfelbaum M, Kohmoto T, DeRosa CM, Smith CR. Histologic appearance of transmyocardial laser channels after 4½ weeks. Ann Thorac Surg 1996;61:1532-1535.
13. Kohmoto T, Fisher PE, Gu A, Zhu SM, Smith CR, Burkhoff D. Physiology of chronic transmyocardial laser channel created with a CO2 laser. Circulation 1995:92 (suppl I):I-176. (abstract)
14. Kohmoto T, Fisher PE, Gu A, Zhu SM, Yano OJ, Spotnitz HM, Smith CR, Burkhoff D. Does blood flow through holmium:YAG transmyocardial laser channels? Ann Thorac Surg 1996;61:861-868.

15. Kohmoto T, Fisher PE, Gu A, Zhu SM, Smith CR, Burkhoff D. Does blood flow through transmyocardial CO_2 laser channels? J Am Coll Cardiol 1996;27:13A. (abstract)

16. Kowallik P, Schulz R, Guth BD, Schade A, Paffhausen W, Gross R, Heusch G. Measurement of regional myocardial blood flow with multiple colored microspheres. Circulation 1991;83:974-982.

17. Whittaker P, Kloner RA, Przyklenk K. Laser-mediated transmural myocardial channels do not salvage acutely ischemic myocardium. J Am Coll Cardiol 1993;22:302-309.

18. Kohmoto T, Fisher PE, DeRosa C, Smith CR, Burkhoff D. Evidence of angiogenesis in regions treated with transmyocardial laser revascularization.

19. Landrenau R, Nawarawong W, Laughlin H, Ripperger J, Brown O, McDaniel W, McKown D, Curtis J. Direct CO_2 laser "revascularization" of the myocardium. Lasers Surg Med 1991;11:35-42.

20. Hardy RI, James FW, Millard RW, Kaplan S. Regional myocardial blood flow and cardiac mechanics in dog hearts with CO_2 laser-induced intramyocardial revascularization. Basic Res Cardiol 1990;85:179-197.

21. Pifarré R, Jasuja ML, Lynch RD, Neville WE. Myocardial revascularization by transmyocardial acupuncture: a physiologic impossibility. J Thorac Cardiovasc Surg 1969;58:424-431.

22. Yano OJ, Bielefeld MR, Jeevanandam V, Treat MR, Marboe CC, Spotnitz HM, Smith CR. Prevention of acute regional ischemia with endocardial laser channels. Ann Thorac Surg 1993;56:46-53.

23. Jeevanandam V, Auteri JS, Oz MC, Watkins J, Rose EA, Smith CR. Myocardial revascularization by laser-induced channels. Surg Forum 1990;41:225-227.

24. Horvath KA, Smith WJ, Laurence RG, Schoen FJ, Appleyard RF, Cohn LH. Recovery and viability of an acute myocardial infarct after transmyocardial laser revascularization. J Am Coll Cardiol 1995;25:528-563.

25. Whittaker P, Rakusan K, Kloner RA. Transmural channels can protect ischemic tissue: Assessment of long-term myocardial response to laser- and needle-made channels. Circulation 1996;93:143-152.

6

POTENTIAL LASER WAVELENGTHS FOR PERCUTANEOUS ENDOMYO-CARDIAL REVASCULARIZATION

Joel D. Eisenberg, On Topaz, George S. Abela
Department of Medicine, Division of Cardiology, Michigan State University, East Lansing, Michigan.

INTRODUCTION

Revascularization of the heart has been extensively investigated in the past fifty years. The primary goal has been to restore blood flow to ischemic areas. Many techniques have been tested; the Vineberg procedure, when the internal mammary artery is implanted directly into the ventricular wall [1,2] (Figure 1); the Beck procedure when the visceral pericardium is irritated to stimulate neovascularization at the epicardial surface [3]; Favalaro's implantation of double internal mammary artery [4] and then direct grafting of coronary arteries by anastomosis with either saphenous bypass grafts or internal mammary arteries [5]; percutaneous interventional procedures pioneered by Gruentzig when a balloon catheter inflated in the coronary lesion, improved lumen size and distal perfusion [6].

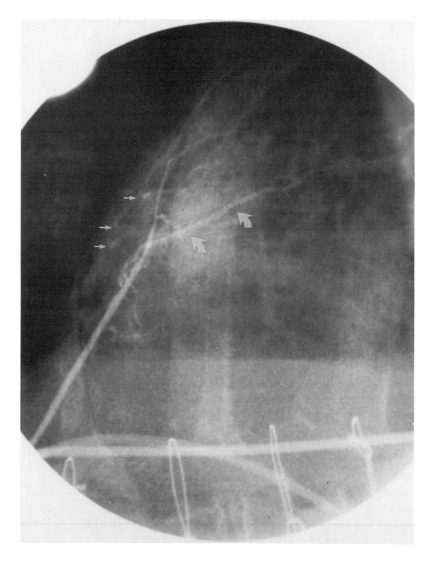

Figure 1. Angiogram of patient with Vineberg graft to the left ventricular wall. Surgery was performed over 20 years prior to this angiography. Right internal mammary artery is seen traveling underneath the LAD (curved arrows) which fills via multiple small collateral branches (small straight arrows) (Topaz et al. Cathet Cardiovasc Diag. Published with permission of authors and publisher).

Over the past several decades, the success of coronary bypass surgery and invasive percutaneous techniques have led to prolonged survival in certain subsets of patients, but mainly in the relief of symptoms in patients with ischemic coronary artery disease [7-11]. These procedures remain primarily palliative. The disease process often continues resulting in the need for additional procedures in many patients at a future date. Large numbers of patients who survive continue to have ischemia, despite earlier revascularization and medical therapy. Diffuse disease may portend a poor outcome for redo coronary bypass surgery or percutaneous angioplasty. This situation calls for an alternative revascularization approach, hence transmyocardial revascularization (TMR) using lasers becomes a highly attractive therapeutic option.

Investigations using laser-made channels for myocardial revascularization were conducted in the early 1980's by Mirhoseini and Drake [12-14, E. Drake, personal communication]. These early studies described the essence of the TMR procedure and have been reconfirmed by subsequent work. Mirhoseini demonstrated the presence of patent transmyocardial channels created by TMR as the major, new source of blood to the ischemic myocardium, while Drake demonstrated neovascularization at the sites of occluded channels. The exact mechanism of myocardial reperfusion by TMR continues to be debated today and conflicting results on outcome and benefits are not yet resolved [15].

The TMR procedure is performed in an open chest preparation using a laser beam directly focused on the epicardial surface of the left ventricle. Channels are made by tunneling from the epicardium through the entire thickness of the myocardial wall into the ventricular chamber. Usually, channels are placed one centimeter apart. By creating multiple channels, the procedure attempts to simulate the reptilian heart physiology, whereby most of the myocardial blood supply comes directly from lacunae within the inner myocardium of the ventricular chamber [16]. The proof of the reptilian heart hypothesis and its correlation to TMR in the human heart has been under intensive investigation and is discussed in other chapters of this book.

The 800-Watt carbon dioxide laser was selected for TMR because of unique tissue effects. By virtue of the high pulse energy, this laser can create a transmyocardial channel in one single pulse. Thus, channels created with this system have minimal thermal injury to the surrounding myocardium. Studies in animals have demonstrated that limitation of thermal injury by creation of clean cut channels result in less tissue scaring and channel closure [17]. Others argue that this mechanism is not essential for the observed benefits of the TMR procedure, therefore, other laser wavelengths may be equally effective, especially if the mechanism of revascularization is attributable to angiogenesis and neovascular growth [E. Drake, personal communication, 18].

To date, more than 3000 patients have been treated worldwide with TMR using the high power carbon dioxide laser (PLC Medical Systems, Franklin, MA). This experience has consistently demonstrated that 71% of the treated patients reported a decrease of at least two classes of angina severity, while control patients who received medical therapy alone had worsening symptoms [19]. Furthermore, studies have shown that TMR treated patients had an improved survival rate. The mortality rate was reported as 6% in the TMR treated group versus 16% in the medically managed group. In 1998, the Food and Drug Administration fully approved the carbon dioxide laser for clinical use. Nevertheless, the reported mortality of TMR via a left chest thoracotomy averages 10% [20]. This may reflect the advanced condition of the patients currently being selected for TMR. Because of the less invasive nature of percutaneous approach, there is a heightened interest in performing TMR via a percutaneous approach [21]. A potential advantage of the percutaneous TMR techniques is its ability to reach the interventricular septum, an area that can not be readily reached by the transthoracic approach.

As for the duration of the channels' patency, studies performed using contrast echocardiography at the Max Plank Institute demonstrated that these channels were still patent at two and the half months following treatment [22]. In two symptomatic patients who underwent concomitant coronary artery bypass surgery, an 800 Watt carbon dioxide laser was used to create TMR channels. One patient received fifteen channels and the other received twenty-five channels. Contrast echocardiography located the channels near the left ventricular apical myocardium extending approximately half way through the thickness of the myocardium. These channels filled in systole only and the contrast washed out after about ten cardiac cycles.

The potential role of TMR in improvement of left ventricular function and volumes in acute ischemia was recently studied in swine by quantitative measurement using an ultrafast 3D magnetic resonance imaging (MRI) technique [23]. The authors concluded that TMR prior to circumflex coronary artery occlusion preserved left ventricular diastolic function and volume. However, a shortcoming of this study was that it did not define the area at risk relative to the area of potential benefit treated by TMR.

Anatomic and physiologic observations following TMR do not always seem to be congruent. Horvath et al studied the effect of TMR with an 800 Watt carbon dioxide laser on the viability and recovery following myocardial infarction in sheep. They demonstrated that in acute infarction created in thirty sheep by occlusion of the left anterior descending coronary artery, the TMR treated group had relatively preserved regional contractility [24]. Moreover, the area of necrosis within the area at increased risk was significantly less (reperfusion group 44 ± 6% and control infarction group 39 ± 5% versus laser group 6 ± 2%). In sheep followed chronically after experimental acute myocardial infarction (thirty days), the TMR group had evidence of myocardial contractility, while the non-TMR group had an akinetic infarcted segment. Histologic analysis demonstrated patent channels at thirty days following TMR.

In another report, Hardy et al demonstrated that laser channels remained patent for two weeks following treatment while needle puncture channels were occluded within forty-eight hours [25]. Studying canine hearts, this group of investigators demonstrated that myocardial perfusion could occur from the left ventricular chamber if the left ventricular pressure was elevated (207 ± 16.1 mm Hg) [14]. Human data seems to be more conflicting. Initial observations made by Mirhoseini reported patent channels following TMR [13,26]. Frazier et al, from the Texas Heart Institute, have corroborated these initial findings demonstrating patent channels in hearts of patients who died three months after TMR [27]. These channels were endothelialized, containing blood cells that suggested functioning channels. However, a more recent report by Gassler et al noted that in four patients who underwent TMR, the channels were fibrosed and occluded at the time of autopsy [18]. Only one of these patients survived the early post-operative period and the others were clearly non-responders to TMR treatment [11]. Krabatsch et al, while also noting closed and fibrosed channels, documented significant neovascularization [28]. These data indicate that the exact mechanism by which TMR perfuses the myocardium and relives angina, reduces ischemia and prolongs survival deserve further investigation.

Efficacy in humans may be validated by improvement in ischemic testing results. Donovan et al noted improvement in wall motion assessed by dobutamine stress echocardiography [29]. Twelve patients who underwent open thoracotomy TMR with a 1000 Watt carbon dioxide laser were assessed pre-operatively and postoperatively at three and six months. They noted overall improvement in wall motion scores that persisted in the nine follow-up patients evaluated at six months. The improvement was more evident in segments that had received TMR. This study, while provocative, will clearly need to be validated in larger numbers of patients. Also, this study appeared to lack blinding of the interpreting physician to the therapy and segments involved.

LASER WAVELENGTHS FOR PERCUTANEOUS
ENDOMYOCARDIAL REVASCULARIZATION (PTER)

The preferable wavelength for use in percutaneous endomyocardial revascularization has not been determined. Thus, further investigation of various wavelengths is warranted. Although some of these wavelengths may have desirable laser-tissue interaction, limitations may be related to laser equipment and delivery systems. The following is a listing of the various laser wavelengths and corresponding experiments describing the effects on myocardial tissue.

Erbium YAG (2,940nm)
The fiber optics required to conduct Er:YAG are specially grown, single, crystal sapphire fibers. These fibers are fragile, but can be coupled efficiently to the laser. However, a major limitation is the radius of bend of the fiber that is a minimum of one and the half inches or greater. This poses some limitations to the flexibility requirements needed for cardiovascular applications.

The advantages of the Er:YAG laser include a clean-cut tissue profile and minimal thermal damage to surrounding tissue. Experiments performed by Abela et al (unpublished) were conducted using sapphire fibers polished on both ends and coupled to an Er:YAG laser (Schwartz Electro-Optics, Orlando, FL). The fibers had a NA of 0.2 and had no cladding. The energy output was adjusted at the fiber tip to be 250 mJ per pulse applied to the tissue surface. This represents 61% transmission of the laser output energy of 415 mJ per pulse over a one-meter long optical fiber.

Experiments were performed on calf heart muscle by positioning the 300 μm core optical fiber tip at 1 mm distance from the tissue surface. Laser irradiation was performed using a dose matrix between 35 mJ and 250 mJ per pulse. A total of sixty pulses were delivered per attempted channel. All the channels were made while dripping a solution of saline on the surface of the tissue to keep the surface moist. In these experiments, the optical fiber was not advanced into the tissue while lasing.

The data revealed that channel depth correlated with laser pulse energy and since each channel was made at a fixed number of pulses (sixty per channel), channel size increased with pulse energy. At the highest pulse energy of 250 mJ per pulse, the average channel depth was 12 mm. At the lowest energy levels (35 mJ) small yet distinct channels could be detected on tissue sectioning.

Histologic analysis of the myocardial channels demonstrated that the pulse energy density used was well above the tissue ablation threshold at the fiber to tissue distances used. Clean cut tissue channels were seen with minimal to absent thermal injury. However, a small zone of tissue desiccation was noted. Minimal tissue dissection and tearing was noted in the walls of the channels (Figure 2).

In a separate group of experiments, the fiber optic was gently advanced into the tissue during laser was activation with 250 mJ per pulse. A full thickness channel was created with a diameter equivalent to the diameter of the optical fiber. Twenty to fifty pulses could penetrate the full thickness of the myocardial wall (1-1.5 cm). Minimal fiber damage was noted during this attempt.

The conclusion of this study is that both contact and non-contact fiber delivery of Er:YAG via sapphire fibers could be used to create clean-cut channels in myocardial tissue. This was accomplished in the presence of a fluid medium, which is highly absorbed by the Er:YAG wavelength at 2,940 nm. Overall, these results are encouraging and suggest that percutaneous endomyocardial laser recanalization may be feasible using the Er:YAG laser.

Holmium:YAG (2,100 nm)
Oesterle et al reported on myocardial channels made by the use of a catheter delivered holmium:YAG laser (CardioGenesis, Sunnyvale, CA) via an optical fiber in canine myocardium [30]. The holmium:YAG laser delivered pulses of 2 J at 17 Hz triggered by the EKG signal. This approach utilized standard fluoroscopy and transesophageal echocardiography to guide the laser catheter within the left ventricular chamber orienting it towards the wall and to observe the results. Left ventricular angiograms were performed demonstrating no evidence for either reduction in myocardial contractility or function. Several channels, measuring 3-5 millimeters in diameter and approximately half way into the left ventricular wall, could be detected. These channels filled with contrast agent during myocardial contraction in systole (Figure 3). Histologic analysis of the myocardial channels demonstrated both thermal necrosis and shock wave dissections (Figure 4).

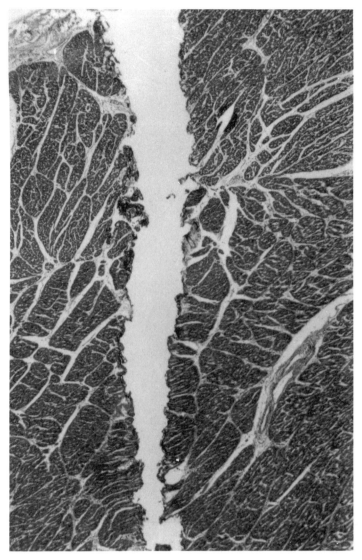

Figure 2. Myocardial channel made by Er:YAG laser using sapphire fiber optics. The energy density was 250 mJ/pulse for a total of 60 seconds. This was done while flushing a solution of normal saline. Minimal thermal injury is noted in the myocardium adjacent to the channel lumen and channel edges are sharp with a few lateral dissection planes from shock wave effects.

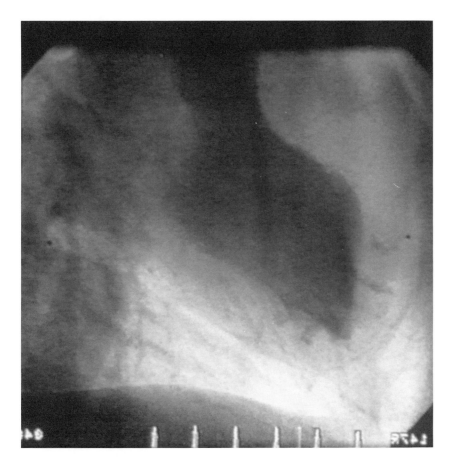

Figure 3. Left ventriculogram in RAO projection in dog. Multiple transmyocardial channels were made in the apex of the left ventricle.

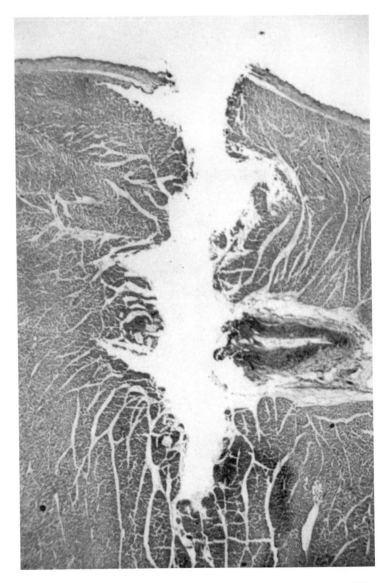

Figure 4. Myocardial channel made by a holmium:YAG laser using a 600 μm core fiber under a saline solution. Both shock wave and some thermal injury can be seen. The laser channel has cut though the edge of an intamyocardial artery (hematoxylin and eosin, original magnification 25X).

To date, reports of this system's performance involved twelve inoperable patients [31]. TMR was performed using a coaxial catheter system enabling a percutaneous approach for access to the endocardium for myocardial revascularization. A steerable laser catheter is advanced through a 9F guide [Figure 5]. Biplane fluoroscopy was used to guide catheter positioning. A 400 μm fiber with a microlens tip was used to focus the laser beam. The holmium:YAG laser was used at a fluence of 83 J/cm² at 30 Hz. Lasing was timed by ECG synchronization. Lesions were created in the endocardial surface to a predesigned depth. An average of ten laser-induced channels was made per patient. Six months post-procedure, follow-up revealed that the angina score was reduced by one to two classes. Complications included one case of tamponade that required percutaneous evacuation.

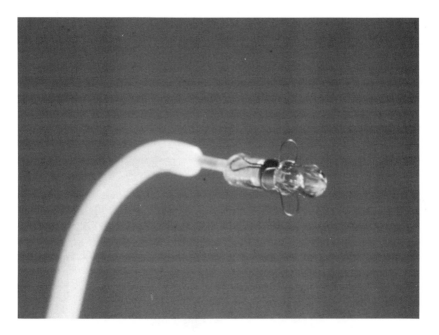

Figure 5. Catheter used to create channels in ventricle. A shielded lens tipped optical fiber is shown extruded from the tip of an introducer catheter. The introducer catheter is rotated around its central axis to reach various positions to contact the left ventricular wall. A winged wire ring around the neck of the fiber optic tip is used to prevent full penetration of the optical system to avoid perforation. (CardioGenesis, Sunnyvale, CA).

Using another holmium:YAG system (Eclipse, Sunnyvale, CA) three patients underwent percutaneous TMR [32]. This system incorporates a multifiber steerable coronary catheter system. TMR performed with the holmium:YAG system in the open chest setting has been reported to have beneficial clinical results comparable to those of the pulsed carbon dioxide TMR system [33].

Argon (488;514 nm)

In 1983, a preliminary study was performed demonstrating the feasibility of laser ablation of atrioventricular (AV) conduction [34,35]. The experiment involved irradiation of the His Bundle in order to create a complete heart block. This was successfully performed in five of six dogs using an optical fiber (coupled to an argon laser) that was extended from the tip of an electrode catheter. AV block was successfully obtained by creation of a myocardial channel in the upper portion of the interventricular septum that cut through the conduction tissues (Figure 6). An associated pathologic feature of this procedure was intramyocardial hematoma formation at some of the irradiated sites [35]. Interestingly, this pathologic feature is similar to that noted with TMR. Recent studies, using an Argon laser delivered with a 600 μm core fiber under saline solution, demonstrated a wedge shaped myocardial channel with surrounding thermal necrosis (Figure 7).

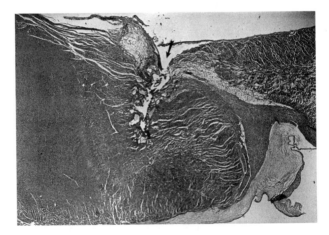

Figure 6. Histologic cross section of crater formed at the tricuspid valve ring. A channel of vaporized myocardial tissue is seen extending about halfway through the interventricular septum below the central fibrous body (arrow). The conduction tissues are also interrupted along this path (hematoxylin and eosin (24X). (From Curtis et al [35], with permission of author and publisher)

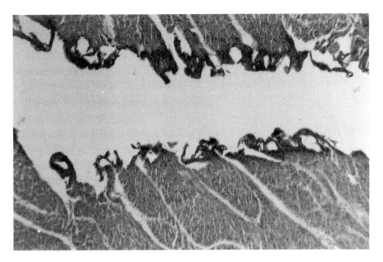

Figure 7. Myocardial channel made by a continuous wave argon ion laser using a 600 μm core silica fiber. Power used was 2 W for 10 seconds with myocardial tissue immersed in saline. Extensive thermal injury is noted on the channel edges. (hematoxylin and eosin, magnification 25X)

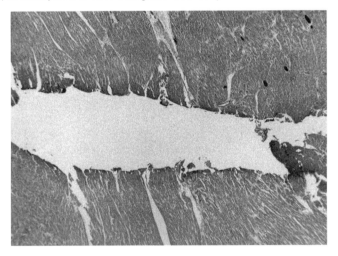

Figure 8. Myocardial channel made using an excimer laser using multifiber optical catheter (Spectranetics, Colorado Springs, CO). The energy density used was 60 mJ/pulse for a total of 2000 pulses with the myocardial tissue immersed in saline.

Excimer (XeCl; 308 nm)
Fresh adult pig hearts from an abattoir were irradiated using a 1.7 French multifiber laser angioplasty catheter (Spectranetics, Inc., Colorado Springs, CO) (Abela et al unpublished data). Lasing was performed by gentle contact of the catheter tip to the myocardial surface with the catheter fixed in place using a micrometer. The experiment was conducted in a normal saline filled tissue bath as described in earlier studies [36]. Laser energy, that was maximal for the excimer laser system used, was set at 60 mJ/pulse for a total of 2000 pulses (25 Hz for 60 seconds). Tissue histology revealed clean edge channels in the myocardium extending approximately 1 cm in depth (Figure 8).

Pulsed Dye Laser (570 nm)
Fresh adult pig hearts from an arbatoir were irradiated using a 600 μm core fiber (Candela flash lamp pulsed dye laser, Candela, MA) (Abela et al, unpublished data). Lasing was performed by gentle contact of the catheter tip to the myocardial surface with the catheter fixed in place using a micrometer (10 Gms). A normal saline filled tissue bath was utilized as described in earlier studies [36]. Maximal laser energy was used at 70 mJ/pulse (10 Hz for 60 seconds). Histologic analysis demonstrated the channel edges to be irregular with residual tissue fragments (Figure 9). Only minimal thermal and shock wave injury were observed. These findings were interpreted as most compatible with incomplete tissue ablation due to insufficient laser energy generated.

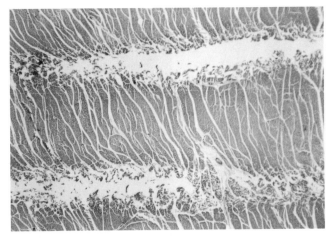

Figure 9. Myocardial channels made using a flash lamp pulsed dye laser at 570 nm coupled to a 600 μm core fiber. The pulse energy was 80 mJ and a total of 480 pulses were delivered. The channels contain extensive tissue fragments.

Diode Laser (805nm/980nm)

In a group of three open chest sheep, *in vivo* laser irradiation of myocardium was performed at 5, 10, 15, and 20 Watts generated from either a Nd:YAG (1064 nm), or 805nm, or 980 nm diode lasers for periods of 60 seconds (Abela et al, unpublished data). Under general anesthesia, sheep hearts were exposed through a median-sternotomy. Laser energies were delivered by a straight 600 μm fiber housed in a catheter held on the beating heart. Saline flush rate was kept at 20 ml/min. Also, myocardial surface temperature was measured by a thermocouple attached to the housing catheter in contact with the heart surface. A total of thirty-nine lesions were created with an average of three lesions for each laser power generated with each laser system.

The greatest central char and tissue vaporization occurred with the 805 nm diode at 15 W and 20 W. There was less char in lesions created by the 980 nm diode laser. Tissue cavitation occurred only occasionally with the 980 nm diode or Nd:YAG lasers 15W and 20W of energy. The decrease in lesion width and penetration depth at 20W of laser power for these lasers indicates that surface tissue carbonization had already occurred within the first few seconds of the 60 second irradiation period. The phenomenon is attributed to the fact that the carbonized surface tissue blocks the entry of laser energy into deeper region of the tissue.

Although the diode laser wavelengths tested may not provide the preferred types of channels needed for such a procedure, this study demonstrates the feasibility of creating diode laser induced tissue injury in myocardium by a percutaneous approach.

CATHETER APPROACHES FOR PERCUTANEOUS ENDOMYOCARDIAL REVASCULARIZATION

The use of an optical fiber in the left ventricle of the heart chamber is not novel. This technology was first developed for treatment of conduction tissue ablation in the myocardium [34,37]. Indeed, performance of TMR as a percutaneous procedure was readily predictable and obvious based upon these early experiments [34,35,37-39]. In fact, the effect on myocardium could be used and interpreted equally for both applications.

Further studies assess the use of laser irradiation of the myocardium for treatment of hypertrophic cardiomyopathy [40]. Two types of devices have been utilized in these early studies. They both include a standard catheter with a central lumen. One is with, and one is without, an electrode at the catheter tip [41]. As previously described for intravascular laser catheter techniques, this catheter is now used to guide the optical fiber in the left ventricular chamber under fluoroscopic guidance and then positioning the catheter at the desired site for laser irradiation (Figure 10).

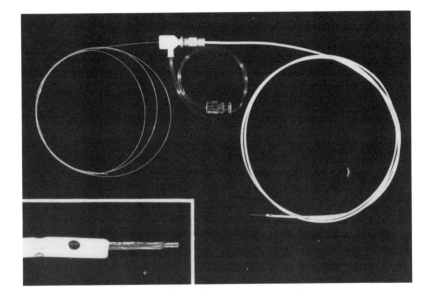

Figure 10. A 200 μm core silica fiber with a metal-tipped marker emerging from the end of a No. 5F catheter (magnified in insert). A hemostasis valve at the hub of the catheter allows for simultaneous injection of contrast media through a side port with the fiber in position for lasing (Abela et al. Circulation. Published with permission of author and publisher).

Potential Side Effects
Early experience with such devices demonstrated that if the optical fiber is advanced into the tissue while lasing, it results in thermal injury regardless of the

wavelength used. Back reflection on the optical fiber tip will turn any laser system primarily into a thermal probe. Furthermore, the advancement of an optical fiber (like any catheter) into cardiac tissue causes myocardial irritability that may induce ventricular arrhythmias [42]. Lastly, there is the possibility of breaking off of an optical fiber in the contracting muscle of the heart leaving a shard of glass. Potentially, it can result in embolization of either glass material or clots that may cause strokes or other organ infarcts. Other possible side effects include the development of an intramyocardial hematoma (Figure 11) and the potential for pain sensation by the patient during the laser channel tunneling [43].

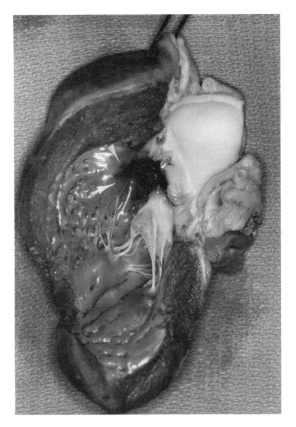

Figure 11. Heart of dog following fifteen laser exposures. Left ventricular chamber with an area of thermal necrosis and hemorrhage (arrow heads) below the aortic valve. No perforation of the septum is noted. (Curtis et al. Pace. Published with permission of author and publisher).

Given the experience with these earlier approaches, modifications were instituted to protect the optical system at the fiber tip in order to preserve optical performance [44]. Also, the use of modified fiber tip lensing systems allows side firing of laser energy relative to the long axis of the catheter tip. Such a system could deliver laser irradiation within the LV without direct tissue contact or penetration of the optical fiber into the myocardium. Further enhancement to the delivery of laser energy to the tissue and to reduce thermal injury includes a jet of saline to clear blood from the laser path. This achieves a more reproducible laser dose treatment effect [43].

The more recent catheter versions have been designed to provide stability within the ventricular chamber. An example is a catheter system with an extendible tip (Figure 12). This catheter was tested in sheep hearts using special side-emitting catheters to deliver laser energies generated from cw Nd:YAG laser (1064 nm) for *in vivo* photocoagulation [45]. The experiment was performed under general anesthesia, whereby the catheter was introduced via a femoral artery cutdown and advanced into the left ventricle of six sheep under fluoroscopic guidance. Laser energies ranging from 100 up to 2400 joules were used to create fifteen circular or elliptical lesions with surface dimensions up to 25 mm x 12 mm and a depth of 9 mm (full LV wall thickness), with a mean lesion size of 9.9 ± 5.2 mm in diameter and 5.8 ± 3.2 mm in depth. A saline flush rate at 20 mL/min was used in all experiments. The outer catheter body acts as an anchor while the inner catheter section acts to probe the free myocardial wall. One advantage is that such a system may allow for precise localization and deposition of laser channels at known distances from each other. Furthermore, the adaptation of a navigation system helps to identify the site of treatment in the myocardium and permits retracing of the various sites visited by the catheter. Navigation can provide the necessary tools for optimal percutaneous endomyocardial revascularization [46].

CorMedica Corp. (Natick, MA) developed a unique technique by incorporating the above steerable catheter to an electromagnetic navigational system. This guided approach allows the user to tracks the ischemic zone of myocardium and provides an endocardial surface map that localizes the site of channels. The system includes a steerable bend, with a deflectable and extendible catheter tip. To stabilize the catheter in a beating heart, the deflectable bend of the catheter is securely positioned in the apex of left ventricle. From this stable site, the mapping and laser portion of the coaxial catheter system can be extended over the full length of the ventricular free wall. This function combined with the rotation of the catheter will provide the important advantage of a full sweep of the endocardial surface with exact localization of the catheter tip.

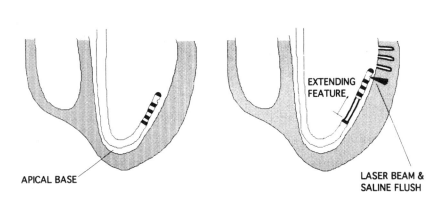

Figure 12. Diagram of catheter delivery system forming a bend at the left ventricular apex to stabilize the system during myocardial contractility (CorMedica, Natick, MA). B. The catheter tip is designed to extend from the apical position to sweep the base of the heart. The laser beam is discharged at right angles to the catheter shaft. The tip can reach the septum, inferior and lateral walls by rotating the base of the catheter. (Wagshall et al. Pace 19; 245).

NEW DEVELOPMENTS

New approaches to deliver laser energy that result in a clean cut tissue edge may be done using a diode laser at the tip of the catheter itself. This may be achieved by pumping a chip at the catheter tip using a pulsed laser. Such a system has the advantage of providing laser energy at the end of the catheter without the loss of beam coherence [47]. Other developments include the introduction of gene codes while creating the laser channel to enhance angiogenesis [48].

SUMMARY

Laser irradiation of the myocardium has been available for over a decade. The effect of laser on the myocardium are well established using various wavelengths and fiber-optic delivery systems. Revived interest has been recently generated by the initial success of surgical TMR in the treatment of ischemia and mainly the symptomatic relief of angina. The logical extension is to deliver laser via a percutaneous approach based on systems which have been available and tested both in the coronary arteries and cardiac chambers. Success and safety in the acute setting, as well as long term benefits need to be demonstrated in future experiments and then in clinical trials. If percutaneous TMR is as successful as the intraoperative approach, then patients who are candidates may benefit without the risk of general anesthesia and thoracotomy. However, the intraoperative and percutaneous approaches could be complementary. Many patients who can be partially revascularized might benefit from TMR to areas of the myocardium that are inoperable at the time of coronary bypass surgery. Those who are not operative candidates could receive PTER. Furthermore, use of PTER as an adjunct to balloon angioplasty would be another likely possibility. Some overlap will exist as in the case of bypass and angioplasty today. These clinical issues should be resolved based upon ongoing refinements in technology, clinical trials, and local expertise in the use of either approach.

References

1. Vineberg A. Development of an anastomosis between the coronary vessels and a transplanted internal mammary artery. Can Med Assoc J 1946;55:117-119.
2. Topaz O, Pavlos S, Nair R, Hsu J. Veinberg procedure revisited: Angiographic evaluation and reoperation 21 years following bilateral internal mammary implantation. Cathet Cardiovac Diagn 1992;25:218-222.
3. Beck CS. The development of a new blood supply to the heart by operation. Ann Surg 1935;102:801-803.
4. Favaloro RG, Effler DB. Double internal mammary artery myocardial implantation: clinical evaluation of results in 150 patients. Circulation 1968;37:549-555.
5. Favaloro RG. The development phase of modern coronary artery surgery. Am J Cardiol 1990;66:1496-1503.
6. Gruentzig AR, Senning A, Siegenthaier WE. Non-Operative dilatation of coronary artery stenosis. Percutaneous transluminal coronary angioplasty. N Engl J Med 1979;301:61.
7. Passamani E, Davis KB, Gillespie MJ, Killip T. A randomized trial of coronary artery bypass surgery: Survival of patients with a low ejection fraction. N Engl J Med 1985;312:1685.
8. The Veterans Administration Coronary Artery Bypass Surgery Cooperative Study Group: Eleven-year survival in the Veterans Administration randomized trial of coronary bypass surgery for stable angina. N Engl J Med 1984;311:1333.
9. Yusuf S, Zucker D, Peduzzi P., et al.: Effect of coronary artery bypass graft surgery on survival: Overview of 10 year results from randomized trials by the Coronary Artery Bypass Graft Surgery Trialists Collaboration. Lancet 1994;344:563.
10. Parisi AF, Folland ED, and Hartigan P. A comparison of angioplasty with medical therapy in the treatment of single-vessel coronary artery disease: Veterans Affairs ACME Investigators. N Engl J Med 1992;326:10.
11. Alderman EL, Fisher LD, Litwin P, Kaiser GC, et al (1983) Results of coronary artery surgery in patients with poor left ventricular function (CASS).
12. Mirhoseini M, Cayton MM. Revascularization of the heart by a laser. J Microsurg 1981;2:253-260.
13. Mirhoseini, M. Mary Cayton. Abela, GS. (Editor) Lasers in Cardiovascular Medicine and Surgery: Fundamentals and Techniques. Martinus Nijhoff, (Kluwer), Boston. 1990.
14. Hardy RI, James FW, Millard RW, Kaplan S. Regional Myocardial blood flow and cardiac mechanics in dog hearts with C02 laser-induced intramyocardial revascularization. Basic Res Cardiol 1990;85:179-197.
15. Topaz O. Laser (Topol ed) Textbook of interventional cardiology. 3rd edition. W.B. Saunders, Philadelphia; 1998: Chapter 32.
16. Lanzafame RJ. "Louisiana Leapers". Editorial. J Clin Laser Med Surg 1997;15:241.
17. Whittaker, P (1997). Transmyocardial laser revascularization-open versus closed channels: what makes the difference? Lasers Surg Med 1997;Suppl 9, 11. (abstract)

18. Gassler N, Wintzer H-O, Stubbe H-M, Wullbrand A, Helmchen U. Transmyocardial Laser Revascularization: Histological Features in Human Nonresponder Myocardium. Circulation 1997;95:371-375.

19. PR Newswire "Food and Drug Administration Says PLC systems can stop randomizing patients to medical management in multicenter TMR clinical trials patents previously randomized to medical management" 09/11/96 13:55:41.

20. Wistow T, Tait S, Sharples L, Caine N et al. (1996) Transmyocardial Revascularization international registry. Cardiostim (10th International Congress) Euro J Card Pacing Electro 1996;6 (suppl 5;1197):300.

21. Rosengart TK. Transmyocardial laser revascularization - a technique in evolution. J Clin Laser Med Surg 1997;15:299-300.

22. Berwing K, Gauer EP, Strasser R, Kolverkorn WP, Bertschmann W. Transmural Laser revascularization: First proof of perfusion through open Laser Channels. German Society of Cardiologists April 1996, Mannheim, Germany.

23. Cayton M, Wang Y, Jerosch-Herold, Klassen C, Unress M, Ugurbil K, Sampson C, Wann SL, Mirhoseini M. Ventricular Function and Volumes in Acute Ischemia after Transmyocardial Laser Revascularization: Quantification by Cine Magnetic Resonance Imaging. Circulation 1996;94:I-295. (abstract)

24. Horvath KA, Smith WJ, Laurence RG, Schoen FJ, et al.. Recovery and viability of an acute myocardial infarct after transmyocardial laser revascularization. J Am Coll Cardiol 1995;25:258-263.

25. Hardy RI, Bove KE, James FW, Kaplan S et al. A histologic study of laser-induced transmyocardial channels. Lasers Surg Med 1987;6:563-573.

26. Mirhoseini M, Cayton MM, Shelgikar S, Fisher JC. Clinical report: laser myocardial revascularization. Lasers Surg Med 1986;6:459-461.

27. Cooley DA, Frazier OH, Kadipasaoglu KA, Pehlivanoglu S, Shannon RL, Angellini P (1994). Transmyocardial laser revascularization: Anatomic evidence of long-term channel patency. Texas Heart Inst J 1994;21:220-224.

28. Krabatsch T, Schaper F, Leder C, Tulsner J, Thalmann U, Hetzer R: Histological findings after transmyocardial laser revascularization. J Card Surg 1996;11:326-321.

29. Donovan L, Landolfo K, Lowe J, Clements F, Coleman R, and Ryan T. Improvement in inducible ischemia during dobutamine stress echocardiography after transmyocardial laser revascularization in patients with refractory angina pectoris. J Am Coll Cardiol 1997;30:607-12.

30. Kim CR, Kesten R, Javier M, Hayase M, et al. Percutaneous Method of Laser Transmyocardial Revascularization. Cath Cardio Diagn 1997;40:223-228.

31. Oesterle SN, Cerhard S, Lauer B, Reifart N, Wolfgang J. (1997) Percutaneous Myocardial Laser Revascularization: Initial Human Experience. Circulation 1997; Suppl I; 1205.

32. IndustryTrak (Business Wire) "First Eclipse percutaneous TMR cases successfully performed. 06/12/97.

33. Almanza O, Wassmer P, Moreno CA, Revall S, et al. Laser Transmyocardial revascularization (LTMR) improves myocardial blood flow via collaterals. J Am

Coll Card 1997;29:99A. (abstract)

34. Abela GS, K, Griffin JC, Hill JA, Normann S, Conti CR. Transvascular Argon Laser-Induced Atrioventricular Conduction Ablation in Dogs. Circulation 1983;68:111-145.

35. Curtis AC, Abela GS, Griffin J, Hill JA, Normann SJ. Transvascular Argon Laser Ablation of Atrioventricular Conduction in Dogs: Feasibility and Morphologic Results. Pace 1989;12:347-357.

36. Friedl SE, Mathews ED, Miyamoto A, Abela GS. Intravascular Ultrasound can be used to Evaluate Pulsed Ho:YAG Laser Ablation of Arterial Tissue. Lasers Surg Med 1995;16:156-163.

37. Lee Ga, Ikeda RM, Teis J, Strobbe D, et al. Effects of laser irradiation delivered by flexible fiberoptic system on the left ventricular internal myocardium. Am Heart J 1983;106:587-590.

38. Abela GS, Conti CR. Laser revascularization: What are its prospects? J Cardiovasc Med 1983;8:977-984.

39. Vincent GM, Fox J, Bendick GA, Hunter J, et al.. Laser catheter ablation of simulated ventricular tachycardia. Lasers Surg Med 1987;7:421-425.

40. Isner JM, Clarke RH, Pandian NG, Donaldson RF, et al. Laser myoplasty for hypertrophic cardiomyopathy: initial in-vitro experience in human postmortem hearts and in-vivo experience in canine model (transarterial) and human patient (intra-operative). Am J Cardiol 1984;53:1620-1626.

41. Abela GS, Normann SJ, Cohen DM, Franzini D, Feldman RL, Crea F, Fenech A, Pepine CJ, Conti CR. Laser Recanalization of Occluded Atherosclerotic Arteries: An In Vivo and In Vitro Study. Circulation 1985;71:403-411.

42. Kadipasaoglu KA, Cihan HB, Clubb FJ, et al. Arrhytmogenic and histologic properties of three laser modalities for transmyocardial laser revascularization. Lasers Surg Med 1997;Suppl 9:12. (abstract)

43. Curtis AB, Vincent GM, Abela GS: Laser Catheter Ablation of Arrhythmias. Lasers in Cardiovascular Medicine and Surgery: Fundamentals and Techniques (Ed. GS Abela) Kluwer Academic Publishers, MA 13:189-200, 1990.

44. Curtis AB, Barbeau GR, Friedl SE, Kunz WF, Mansour M, Abela GS. Modification of AV Conduction using a Percutaneous Combined Laser-Electrode Catheter. Pace 1994;17:337-348.

45. Wagshall AB, Weiner BH, Bowden R, Lin FC, Mathews ED, Flynn K, Hennigan C, Huang S-KS, Abela GS. A novel Catheter design for laser photocaogulation of the myocardium to ablate ventricular tachycardia. Pace 1996;19:245. (abstract)

46. Abela GS, Bowden RW (1998) U.S. Patent No. 5,769,843 Percutaneous Endomyocardial Revascularization.

47. Abela GS, Maruska HP (1997) U.S. Patent No. 5,620,439 Catheter and Technique for endovascular myocardial revascularization.

48. Ulrich F, Canto E, Abela GS. Heat shock increases in vitro gene transfection into bovine aorta smooth muscle cells. Lasers Med Surg 1995;Suppl 7:12. (abstract)

7

INITIAL USE OF AN ULTRAVIOLET LASER FOR TMR

Peter Whittaker, Kalin Spariosu,[1] Zonh-Zen Ho[2]

The Heart Institute, Good Samaritan Hospital and Department of Medicine, University of Southern California, Los Angeles, [1]Rockwell Science Center, Thousand Oaks, and [2]Physical Optics Corporation, Torrance, CA.

INTRODUCTION

Although many of the published TMR clinical reports are encouraging [1-3], the procedure remains controversial, primarily because the mechanism of the reported clinical improvement is unknown. Previous work demonstrated that transmural channels made in sheep hearts with an excimer laser [4] and in rat hearts with a hypodermic syringe needles [5] stayed open for at least one month, and in the case of the needle channels, provided protection against subsequent coronary artery occlusion. Nevertheless, these results are in sharp contrast to the closed channels found after holmium:YAG and carbon dioxide laser treatment in dog and pig hearts [6-8]. Our explanation for these conflicting data was that channels remain patent only if injury to tissue surrounding the channels is small; a feature not often reported after channel-making with infrared lasers such as the holmium:YAG and carbon dioxide.

The relatively small amount of damage to surrounding tissue caused by the excimer laser (λ=308 nm) was probably achieved because the mechanism of tissue ablation, direct photon absorption by covalent bonds rather than the water absorption mechanism of infrared laser energy, is conducive to minimizing thermal injury [9]. If this is the case, then other ultraviolet lasers might also be expected to be capable of producing open channels. We therefore examined the ability of a frequency-tripled neodymium:YAG laser ($\lambda = 355$ nm) to create open channels.

The needle method appeared to be successful because the trauma associated with its insertion caused only a thin band of muscle necrosis [5]. However, needle-made channels were found to be much narrower than the diameter of the needle used to create them when examined two months later. This probably occurred because no tissue was extracted at the time of channel-making and therefore, when the needle was removed, the channel diameter immediately decreased because of tissue recoil. To maintain a greater initial channel diameter, we proposed using a hot needle. Other studies have found that tissue stiffness increases after heating [10], and so we speculated that the thermal effect of a hot needle would confer stiffness and rigidity to the channel wall and hence potentially limit the initial tissue recoil.

We therefore tested two different energy doses of the frequency-tripled neodymium:YAG laser and the hot needle method in rat hearts. Channels were made 51-165 days before applying an ischemic challenge in the form of a coronary artery occlusion, with efficacy assessed by measurement of infarct size.

METHODS

Laser Description
We used a pulsed neodymium:YAG laser to create the channels (Laser Photonics, Orlando, FL). The wavelength of this laser is 1064 nm; however, when the beam passes through a crystal to generate the third harmonic, the frequency of the light is tripled such that the resulting light is in the ultraviolet part of the electromagnetic spectrum ($\lambda = 355$ nm). A Q-switch was used, which resulted in a short pulse width (9 ns). We used two doses; a low dose of 5-6 mJ per pulse and a high dose of 9-10 mJ per pulse. These doses were selected on the basis of in vitro experiments in which the laser was used to make channels in pieces of canine myocardium. These pilot experiments revealed doses that were capable of creating

channels surrounded by relatively small amounts of thermal injury. The pulse frequency used was 20 Hz, and the laser beam was focused into optic fibers with a diameter of 400 μm and 600 μm.

Needle Preparation
Hypodermic syringe needles (diameter 400 μm) were placed in a water bath heated to 75-80°C. The needles were attached to syringes so that they could be readily removed from the bath and then immediately used to make a channel.

Channel-making Surgery
Female, retired-breeder Sprague-Dawley rats were anesthetized by intraperitoneal injection of a mixture of ketamine and xylazine, intubated, and ventilated with room air. A thoracotomy was performed through the fifth intercostal space to expose the middle and apical portions of the left ventricle. Six transmural channels were made in the region of the left ventricle perfused by the left coronary artery. Transmural penetration of the channel was confirmed by pulsatile bleeding from the channel of oxygenated blood.

Ischemic Challenge
Two to five months after the initial channel making, the rats were reanesthetized (route and dose as described above). We performed a tracheostomy and ventilated the lungs with room air. The chest was opened through the fourth intercostal space to expose the basal portion of the heart. To occlude the left coronary artery, which lies below the surface of the myocardium, a stitch was taken through the myocardium with a C-1 taper needle and 5-0 polypropylene suture from the atrioventricular groove to the region of the pulmonary cone. Additional sutures were tied to each arm of the stitch suture to allow release of the occlusion knot [11]. A single knot was then tied in the stitch suture to occlude the artery. Limb lead L_1 of the ECG was monitored throughout the experiment and recorded on a chart recorder. After ninety minutes, the occlusion was released by untying the knot. At the end of the 4½ hour reperfusion period, the artery was briefly reoccluded and 0.5 mL of blue pigment (Unisperse Blue, Ciba Geigy Corp.) was injected into the circulation through the left femoral vein. The area not perfused by the occluded artery will appear blue, while the tissue perfused by the artery (referred to as the area at risk) will appear pale. Approximately fifteen seconds after injection of the pigment, with the animal under deep anesthesia, 3 mL of potassium chloride solution was injected into the heart to induce cardiac arrest. The hearts were excised and cut into 4-5 slices parallel to the atrioventricular groove and photographed. The slices were then incubated in a solution of

triphenyltetrazolium chloride (TTC) for 10 minutes at 37°C and rephotographed. With TTC incubation, viable myocardium stains red, while necrotic myocardium does not stain and so appears pale. We used planimetry to measure the size of the area at risk (which was expressed as a percent of the area of the left ventricle), and also the area of necrosis (which was expressed as a percent of both the left ventricle and the area at risk). These results were compared with a complete cohort of historical controls (n=8) from a previous TMR study in our laboratory.

Histologic Analysis
Each of the heart slices was serial sectioned at a thickness of 7 μm and the slides stained with hematoxylin and eosin or picrosirius red [12]. The latter stains muscle yellow and collagen red and was used to identify the channels. To classify a channel as patent, we had to locate a connection to the left ventricular cavity and/or blue pigment within the channel. Fisher et al demonstrated that segments of the original channel can remain open even when there was no open connection to the LV chamber [6,13]. We considered the presence of pigment within the channel equivalent to an LV chamber connection because the rat heart's lack of a native collateral circulation means that the pigment would not be found within the channels unless it had come directly from the LV chamber. The maximum width of fibrosis associated with each channel or channel-remnant was measured with a calibrated eye-piece reticle. The structural organization of collagen in the channel-associated fibrosis was examined using polarized light microscopy. The optical properties of collagen fibers observed with polarized light can be used to assess their two-dimensional orientation [14].

We also measured the collagen content of the myocardium. This was done from polarized light examination of picrosirius red stained sections with a previously published video-image analysis method [15]. Measurements were made in three regions of the intraventricular septum and in three regions of the LV free-wall, remote from any channels.

RESULTS

Mortality
No rats died after channels were made with a hot needle; however, there were four deaths in the low-dose laser group and one in the high dose laser group. All of the deaths occurred within 24 hours of the initial surgery. We did not attempt to determine the cause of death. It is possible that bleeding from open channels persisted leading to hemothorax or there may have been myocardial infarction if

a channel perforated a major coronary artery. However, there is some mortality associated with thoracotomy and so the deaths may be unrelated to the laser treatment. One rat in the low dose laser group was excluded from analysis because of a technical problem with pigment perfusion to delineate the area at risk. Thus, all analysis was carried out on three hearts with the low dose laser, and five with the high dose laser. The lack of any success with the hot needle treatment resulted in the examination of only two animals.

Area at Risk and Infarct Size
The size of the area at risk, expressed as a percent of the left ventricle did not differ between groups (Table 1). In contrast, the area of necrosis, expressed either as a percent of the left ventricle (Table 1) or as a percent of the area at risk (Figure 1), was significantly lower in the high dose laser-treated hearts than in any of the other groups, and the infarcts in this group were patchy and never transmural. Although there were no statistically significant differences amongst the other groups, we did see evidence of local protection in all of the low dose laser-treated hearts. In some slices from these hearts, there were bands of red-staining tissue (i.e., viable muscle) extending radially across the wall within the area at risk (Figure 2). Such TTC staining patterns are not seen in control hearts in which the infarcts are homogeneous and transmural rather than patchy. In the example illustrated in Figure 2, the band of red-staining tissue corresponded to the location of an open channel. The infarcts in the hot needle treated hearts were confluent and transmural.

Table 1. Area at risk and infarct size

	hot needle	low dose laser	high dose laser	control
AR/LV (%)	56±6	53±2	55±4	46±2
AN/LV (%)	35±1	30±1	13±3*	27±3

* P < 0.05 versus all of the other groups

AR/LV - area at risk expressed as a percent of the area of the left ventricle
AN/LV - area of necrosis expressed as a percent of the area of the left ventricle

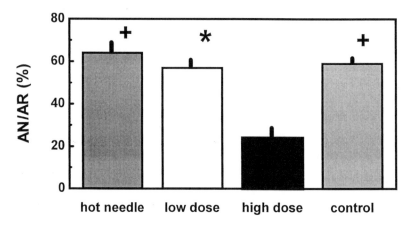

Figure 1. Area of muscle necrosis (AN) expressed as a percent of the area at risk (AR). Infarct size was significantly smaller in the high dose laser group than in any of the other groups (*P<0.01, + P<0.001).

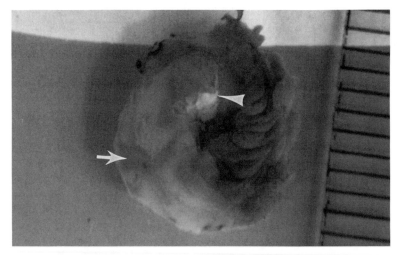

Figure 2. Triphenyltetrazolium chloride stained heart slice from a low dose laser-treated heart. Viable myocardium appears red (dark), while necrotic muscle appears pale. There is a transmural band of viable muscle (arrow) in the center of the necrotic region. On histologic analysis, we found an open channel at this location. Infarcts in untreated hearts subjected to the same duration of ischemia are always confluent and transmural. The bright white region in the subendocardium (arrowhead) is fibrosis associated with another channel.

Electrocardiogram Analysis

Figure 3 shows the relative average amplitude of the Q-waves and the RST complex measured in lead L_1 at the end of the experiment. Q-waves were seen in all cases; however, they were small in the high dose group. In fact, their depth was less than the height of the RST complex (P=0.018) in this group. In contrast, the Q-wave was the most prominent feature in the other two groups. These findings are consistent with the smaller infarcts found in the high dose laser group.

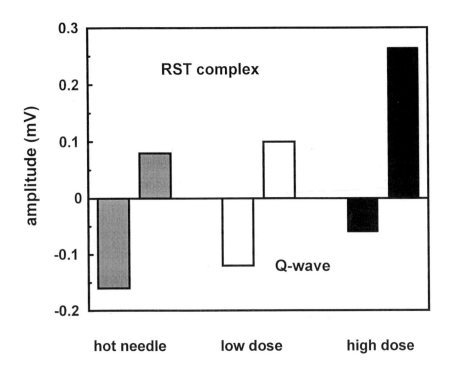

Figure 3. Bar graph showing the mean amplitudes of the Q-wave and RST-complexes in the three groups measured from lead L_1 six hours after coronary artery occlusion. Only in the high dose laser group did the height of the RST complex exceed the depth of the Q-waves. This observation is consistent with the finding of smaller, non-transmural infarcts in the high dose laser group.

Histologic Analysis

We were able to identify 60% of the channels that were originally made. The channels, or their remnants, were readily identified because they were surrounded by scar tissue and extended radially across the wall. The lack of a smooth muscle layer in these structures, in addition to their location, prevented them from being confused with intramyocardial arteries, which were often of a similar size.

There was a significantly higher proportion of open channels found in the high dose group (89%; P<0.05 versus other groups) than in either the low dose (46%) or the hot needle group, where only one open channel was found. The maximum diameter of these open channels did not differ between the two laser groups (high dose = 33 ± 5 μm; low dose = 36 ± 11 μm). The one open hot needle channel was only 8 μm wide. The widest channel found had a maximum diameter of 140 μm (this was in the low dose laser group). We observed blue pigment within the channels and in tissue surrounding the channels in all laser-treated hearts. In contrast, blue pigment was never seen within the area at risk of the hot needle treated hearts. Small vessels were also seen connecting with laser-made channels, which appeared to be capillaries (i.e., they did not possess a medial layer of smooth muscle cells). Examples of open channels with vessels branching off from them are shown in Figures 4 and 5. Blue pigment was be seen within the channel in Figure 5 and within a blood vessel adjacent to the channel. Examination of hematoxylin and eosin stained sections revealed that these channels and the vessels connected to the channels were lined by hematoxylin-positive cell nuclei, which had an appearance consistent with endothelial cells (for example, the cell nuclei projected into the lumen). However, because we were unable to obtain a specific antibody for rat endothelial cells that stained this formalin fixed tissue, this observation remains preliminary and requires confirmation.

The maximum width of channel-associated fibrosis for both open channels and channel remnants is shown in Figure 6 for the three groups. The width of fibrosis was significantly less in the high dose laser group (145 ± 10 μm) than in either the low dose laser (220 ± 24 μm; P<0.05), or the hot needle group (272 ± 46 μm; P<0.01). When the high dose laser group was divided on the basis of the diameter of the optic fiber used, there was no difference in fibrosis width (400μm fiber, 148 ± 13 μm, n = 10; 600 μm fiber, 143 ± 13 μm, n = 8). Similar subgroup analysis revealed no differences in the low dose laser group.

The collagen fibers adjacent to open channels appeared to be aligned predominantly parallel to the direction of the channel; that is radially across the thickness of the ventricular wall. In contrast, in closed channels the collagen fibers were aligned perpendicular to the original channel direction (Figure 7).

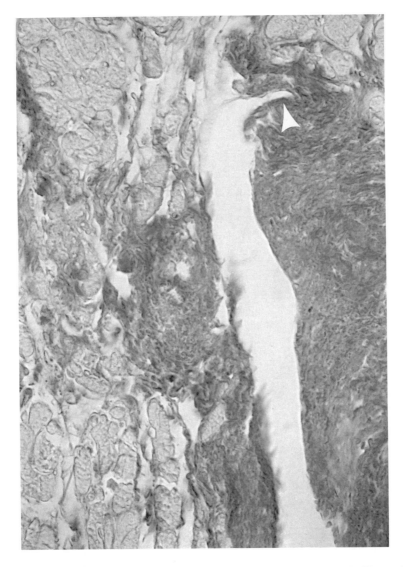

Figure 4. Picrosirius red stained section from the heart slice shown in Figure 2. This open channel was located in the area of TTC positive stained myocardium. The width of the channel is approximately 40 μm. A vessel can be seen connected perpendicular to the direction of the channel (arrowhead). The dark staining material surrounding the channel is fibrosis.

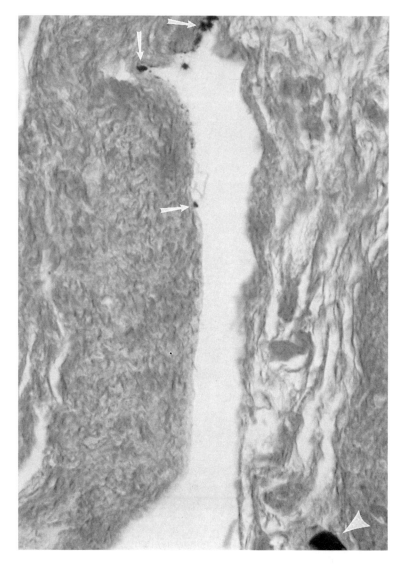

Figure 5. Open channel (45 μm in diameter) containing blue pigment (arrows). Pigment can also be seen in a blood vessel next to the channel (arrowhead). This channel was surrounded by more fibrosis than the channel in Figure 4.

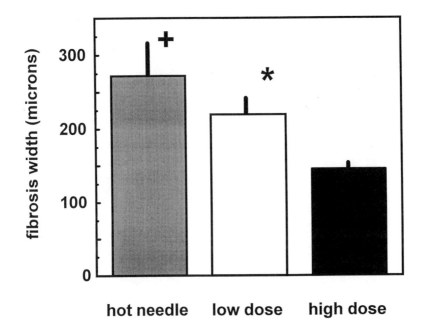

Figure 6. The width of channel-associated fibrosis for all channels or channel remnants identified in each treatment group. The width of fibrosis was significantly less in the high dose laser group than in the other two (* P<0.05, + P<0.01 versus high dose laser treatment).

Collagen Concentration
In the two high dose rats that were followed for approximately 5 months, there was a noticeable increase in collagen concentration in myocardium remote from channels (Figure 8). This increase came from both an increase in the amount of interstitial fibrosis and an increase in fiber thickness. The concentration was significantly higher (6.0 ± 0.7%; P < 0.05) than that in the high dose group followed for two months (3.6 ± 0.6%). Intermediate values were found in the hot needle (4.7 ± 0.3%) and low dose groups (4.2 ± 0.3%).

DISCUSSION

We found that transmural channels can protect against later coronary artery occlusion, but only if the channels remained open and were surrounding by a

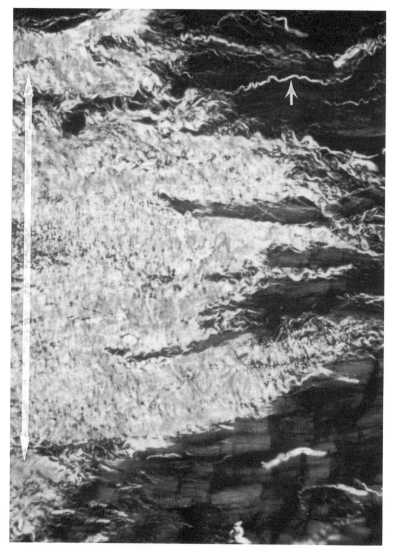

Figure 7. (A) Closed channel. The original channel direction is marked by the large arrow (in the direction from the top to the bottom of the page). The collagen fibers (which appear bright) in the channel-associated scar tissue were aligned perpendicular to the original channel direction (an individual fiber bundle adjacent to the bulk of the scar is marked with the small arrow). Section stained with picrosirius red and viewed with polarized light.

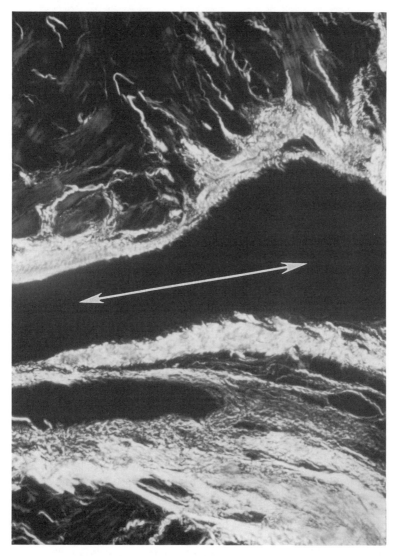

Figure 7. (B) Open channel. The collagen fibers immediately adjacent to the open channel were aligned parallel to the direction of the channel (marked by the arrow).

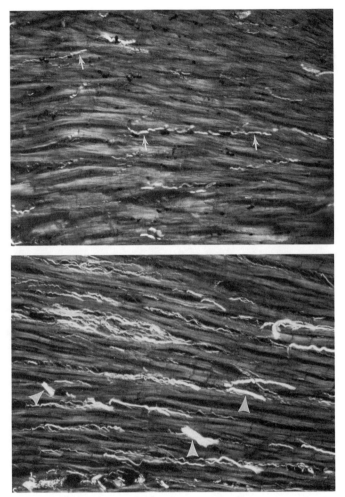

Figure 8. Micrographs from the interventricular septum of rats from the high-dose laser treated group stained with picrosirius red and viewed with circularly polarized light. The collagen fibers appear bright (arrows). The upper panel is from a heart examined two months after channel making. The average collagen concentration in the septum of this heart was 2.5%. The lower panel is from a heart examined five months after channel making with an average collagen concentration of 6.0%. The increase appears to derive primarily from an increase in interstitial fibrosis; however, there also appears to be an increase in the diameter of some fibers (arrowheads).

small band of scar tissue. We propose that open channels are necessary for blood to flow from a region where it is in abundance (the cavity of the left ventricle) to a region where it is absent (the tissue served by the occluded artery), with vascular connections to the channel providing a conduit to the adjacent tissue. However, if there is a large band of scar tissue adjacent to the channel, then these vascular connections will terminate within the scar and never reach the desired target - the surrounding muscle. Thus, excessive fibrosis presents a barrier to useful blood flow (that is, blood flow to muscle). The results of this current study are consistent with our previous studies in which, no matter what channel making method was used, large amounts of channel fibrosis were associated with closed channels and failure to protect against an ischemic challenge [5,15].

Open Versus Closed Channels
The width of fibrosis surrounding each channel, or channel remnant, appeared to be a factor in determining the outcome in our experiments. The group with the largest amount of channel-associated fibrosis, the hot needle-treated group, contained only one open channel and showed no evidence of protection against coronary artery occlusion. The low dose laser group had a patency rate of approximately 50%, but showed only localized evidence of protection against the ischemic challenge. This group was associated with an intermediate amount of fibrosis. The high-dose laser group had the least amount of fibrosis, a 90% patency rate, and a significant amount of protection against ischemia. Thus, there appeared to be a relationship between the width of fibrosis and channel patency; the greater the width of fibrosis, the smaller the likelihood of patency. Nevertheless, the amount of channel-associated fibrosis may not be the only feature of the scar associated with channel patency. However, before discussing this, it is useful to consider what happens to scar tissue during the healing response to the injury caused by channel-making.

The amount of muscle necrosis caused by the initial channel-making procedure will be reflected by the width of channel-associated fibrosis found several months later. Nevertheless, the correlation between initial necrosis and final amount of fibrosis is unlikely to be linear. This is because scars are not passive structures, but possess the ability to contract. However, this is not the rhythmic contraction of cardiac muscle, but rather a slow and progressive contraction mediated by both fibroblasts and actin filament-containing myofibroblasts that reduces the volume of the scar over time. Fisher and colleagues found that although the initial amount of muscle necrosis associated with TMR channels made with a holmium:YAG laser was significantly greater that associated with the use of a carbon dioxide laser, the size of the scar measured six weeks later was similar [13]. Measurements made at two weeks after channel-making, showed that the volume reduction occurred in the scars produced by both lasers; however, the degree of shrinkage was greater in the holmium:YAG scars. Their results may indicate that the greater the initial injury, the greater the subsequent contraction. Such scar contraction may also play a role in channel closure. In fact, channels made in animal hearts with both holmium:YAG and carbon dioxide lasers have been invariably found to have closed after two weeks [6,7]. We speculate that the channel patency found in our study reflects, in part, less initial myocardial necrosis than was caused by the infrared lasers used by Fisher and colleagues. Nevertheless, as mentioned, there are undoubtedly other factors involved in the process of channel closure. For example, the finding of differences in the architecture of collagen fibers within the channel-associated scars between open and closed channels. The exact significance of this finding is unknown. It is possible that the alignment of collagen fibers parallel to the channel direction allows channels to stay open. On the other hand, it is equally possible that this particular structure develops because the channels are open. Clearly, further work is needed to determine what is "cause" and what is "effect".

Even though the high dose laser treatment was successful in limiting infarct size, we observed a marked increase in collagen concentration in the myocardium remote from the channels (Figure 7). This increase was similar to that previously reported after holmium:YAG TMR in rat hearts [5]. Although collagen concentration is known to increase with age in rat hearts, the apparent doubling of collagen concentration in only three months is more than would be expected on the basis of age alone. Thus, it is possible that such myocardial remodeling is a consequence of the laser treatment. The stimulus for the increase is unknown, but the effect illustrates that there may be deleterious consequences of channel making that extend to other regions of the heart, and emphasizes the need for long-term, rather than acute study in TMR protocols.

Mechanical Versus Laser-made Channels
Our hypothesis for using a hot needle may still be valid; however, the needle we used in these experiments was probably too hot. The high temperature appeared to result in more necrosis than the laser treatment and hence a greater amount of scar tissue. The ability to achieve the desired channel configuration with a lower temperature needle has yet to be tested. Although some of the laser-created

channels were able to protect against coronary artery occlusion, it is possible that these channels were not created solely by an ablative process. If the energy was expressed in terms of fluence rather than pulse energy , we found no correlation with infarct size, patency, channel diameter, or fibrosis. The inability to explain our data in terms of fluence values could indicate that this parameter was only one of several that were important. Similarly, the data did not appear to be determined by fiber diameter. The latter would appear to rule out a purely mechanical mechanism for channel creation; that is, the channels were not made by just pushing the fiber through the myocardium. Instead, we raise the possibility that the channels were made by a combination of ablation and mechanical effects; that is the frequency-triple Nd:YAG laser may have acted as a hot needle with the ability to ablate some tissue. This is consistent with the knowledge that ablation efficiency at a wavelength of 355 nm is not as great as at 308 nm. The combination of ablation and mechanical contributions to channel making will always be a possibility when the fiber is manually advanced, but could be eliminated (if necessary) by an automated rate of advancement calculated to permit ablation in front of the advancing fiber.

Limitations

Four limitations of the current study must be acknowledged; (1) the small sample size, (2) the use of rat hearts, (3) the challenge of coronary artery occlusion in a normal heart does not duplicate the intended clinical application of TMR, and (4) there is no direct evidence for blood flow through the channels.

(1) Although the sample sizes in the hot needle and low dose laser groups were small, we have confidence in the conclusions drawn because the data provided was either consistent with previous work or, was consistently reproducible. For example, the infarct size in the hot needle group was very close to that of the control group. In addition, the large width of fibrosis found in the hot needle treated hearts was similar in magnitude to that found in other studies in which there was no reduction in infarct size. Furthermore, the observation of bands of viable muscle in the low dose laser group was consistent and represents such an unusual staining pattern that it is unlikely to be a false positive.

(2) The rat model has been criticized because of the small size of the heart. However, it should be remembered that red blood cells, capillaries, and muscle cells are of similar dimensions in rat and human hearts and therefore the mechanisms of blood flow and oxygen supply will also be similar. Although there

are undoubtedly some scaling issues that may confound direct extrapolation of our results to human hearts, the questions of what should the initial channel diameter be and how many channels should be made have yet to be examined in a systematic fashion in any study; rat or human. It is interesting to note that nine open channels reported from a human autopsy case three months after channel-making with a carbon dioxide laser were 20-75μm wide [16], very close to the diameters reported here. The spot size, and hence the purported initial channel diameter, in this clinical example was 1 mm.

(3) TMR is intended as a treatment for patients with angina refractory to other treatments and to improve perfusion to so-called hibernating myocardium, where muscle is viable but not contracting. There is currently no animal model that adequately duplicates the human disease (as discussed in Chapter 4), and so any animal model used to examine TMR could be termed "inappropriate". Our choice of a challenge of acute myocardial ischemia is severe and would be at the extreme end of what patients might experience. Nevertheless, it is a challenge with a well-defined end-point; infarct size. The lack of an adequate animal model also means that channels are made in normal healthy animal hearts rather than diseased tissue. It is likely that the laser parameters required to create channels will be different in diseased tissue; for example, diseased hearts will probably contain more fibrosis which might mean that more energy will be required to make the channels. Again, these are issues that have yet to be examined in a systematic fashion in any study. The ability to create channels that remain open in a normal healthy animal hearts does, at least, provide some evidence that open channels are possible in human hearts.

(4) The reduction in infarct size and the finding of pigment within the channels and in tissue surrounding the channels represent indirect, rather than conclusive, evidence for blood flow through the channels. Direct documentation of flow will be required before TMR can attain acceptance as a legitimate therapy. So far, in the human trials, the evidence for flow through the channels has been somewhat equivocal [1,3]. However, if, as a significant proportion of the published autopsy cases suggest, the channels are closed [17,18], then flow through such channels is a moot point. The issue of whether or not there is flow through the channels is without doubt the most important question in TMR and will require further examination in appropriately designed animal and clinical studies.

SUMMARY

We have demonstrated that not only are open channels with connections to the left ventricular cavity required to protect against the challenge of acute coronary artery occlusion, but also the channels must be surrounded by a limited amount of scar tissue. We propose that excessive scar tissue provides a barrier that prevents, or severely limits, the amount of blood able to reach muscle cells beyond the zone of fibrosis. In addition, the structural organization of the collagen fibers within the fibrosis may be involved in determining channel patency.

Acknowledgment
This work was supported by a grant from the National Institutes of Health. We thank Seda Dzhandzhapanyan for assistance in the preparation of the histological samples.

References

1. Frazier OH, Cooley DA, Kadipasaoglu KA, Pehlivanoglu S, Lindenmeir M, Barasch E, Conger JL, Wilansky S, Moore WH. Myocardial revascularization with laser. Preliminary findings. Circulation 1995;92[suppl II]:58-65.

2. Donovan CL, Landolfo KP, Lowe JE, Clements F, Coleman RB, Ryan T. Improvement in inducible ischemia during dobutamine stress echocardiography after transmyocardial laser revascularization in patients with refractory angina pectoris. J Am Coll Cardiol 1997;30:607-612.

3. Horvath KA, Cohn LH, Cooley DA, Crew JR, Frazier OH, Griffith BP, Kadipasaoglu K, Lansing A, Mannting F, March R, Mirhoseini MR, Smith C. Transmyocardial laser revascularization: results of a multicenter trial with transmyocardial laser revascularization used as sole therapy for end-stage coronary artery disease. J Thorac Cardiovasc Surg 1997;113:645-654.

4. Mack CA, Magovern CJ, Hahn RT, Sanborn T, Lanning L, Ko W, Isom OW, Rosengart TK. Channel patency and neovascularization after transmyocardial revascularization using an excimer laser. Results and comparisons to nonlased channels. Circulation 1997; 96[suppl II]:II-65-II-69.

5. Whittaker P, Rakusan K, Kloner RA. Transmural channels can protect ischemic tissue. Assessment of long-term myocardial response to laser- and needle-made channels. Circulation 1996;93:143-152.

6. Kohmoto T, Fisher PE, Gu A, Zhu SM, Yano OJ, Spotnitz HM, Smith CR, Burkhoff D. Does blood flow through holmium:YAG transmyocardial laser channels? Ann Thorac Surg 1996;61:861-868.

7. Kohmoto T, Fisher PE, Gu A, Zhu SM, DeRosa CM, Smith CR, Burkhoff D. Physiology, histology, and 2-week morphology of acute transmyocardial channels made with a CO_2 laser. Ann Thorac Surg 1997;63:1275-1283.

8. Fleischer KJ, Goldschmidt-Clermont PJ, Fonger JD, Hutchins GM, Hruban RH, Baumgartner WA. One-month histologic response of transmyocardial laser channels with molecular intervention. Ann Thorac Surg 1996;62:1051-1058.

9. Hartman RA, Whittaker P. The physics of transmyocardial laser revascularization. J Clin Laser Med Surg 1997;15:255-259.

10. Kang T, Resar J, Humphrey JD. Heat induced changes in the mechanical behavior of passive coronary arteries. J Biomech Eng 1995;117:86-93.

11. Himori N, Matsuura A. A simple technique for occlusion and reperfusion of coronary artery in conscious rats. Am J Physiol 1989;256:H1719-H1725.

12. Sweat F, Puchtler H, Rosenthal SI. Sirius red F3BA as a stain for connective tissue. Arch Pathol 1964;78:69-72.

13. Fisher PE, Kohmoto T, De Rosa C, Smith C, Burkhoff D. Natural history of transmyocardial laser revascularization channels: comparison of CO2 and HO:YAG lasers. Lasers Surg Med Suppl 1997;9:11-12. (abstract)

14. Whittaker P, Kloner RA, Boughner DR, Pickering JG. Quantitative assessment of myocardial collagen with picrosirius red staining and circularly polarized light. Basic Res Cardiol 1994;89:397-410.

15. Whittaker P, Kloner RA. Transmural channels as a source of blood flow to ischemic myocardium? Insight from the reptilian heart. Circulation 1997;95:1357-1359.
16. Cooley DA, Frazier OH, Kadipasaoglu KA, Pehlivanoglu S, Shannon RL, Angelini P. Transmyocardial laser revascularization. Texas Heart Inst J 1994;21:220-224.
17. Burkhoff D, Fisher PE, Apfelbaum M, Kohmoto T, DeRosa CM, Smith CR. Histologic appearance of transmyocardial laser channels after 4½ weeks. Ann Thorac Surg 1996;61:1532-1535.
18. Gassler N, Wintzer HO, Stubbe HM, Wullbrand A, Helmchen U. Transmyocardial laser revascularization. Histological features in human nonresponder myocardium. Circulation 1997;95:371-375.

8

THE FIRST CLINICAL TMR TRIAL:
Historical Perspective

John R. Crew
San Francisco Heart Institute at Seton Medical Center, Daly City, CA.

INTRODUCTION

Transmyocardial revascularization (TMR) with a high power carbon dioxide laser began as a sole therapy for coronary artery disease in January 1990 at Seton Medical Center in Daly City, California. The concept and principles for this treatment were derived from the experimental canine and clinical studies done by Mirhoseini. The anatomical model used as the basis for the procedure was the reptilian heart described by Sen. The distinctive features of such hearts, their numerous sinusoids and a relatively limited (versus mammalian hearts) coronary arterial system, have been illustrated by several investigators. In 1988, after careful evaluation of the available data, we agreed that there was enough evidence to believe that we could proceed with the concept of attempting to duplicate the structure of a reptile heart by creating channels through the myocardium.

However, the problem of how to develop a laser with sufficient power to penetrate the wall of a warm, moving heart remained. Prior to this, Mirhoseini performed adjunctive studies using an underpowered carbon dioxide laser to slowly (over approximately 2-3 seconds) penetrate a cold, arrested heart with a 1 mm diameter beam producing a 1 mm diameter channel during cardiopulmonary bypass. Histological evidence of thermal trauma extended only 100 μm from the channel. Autopsy results in one TMR-treated patient who died of cancer 4½ years later revealed patent channels lined with normal endothelium. Since then Cooley and Frazier reported another clinical case indicating the same findings.

THE FIRST PATIENT

In 1988, we obtained our first carbon dioxide laser from Laser Engineering (LEI) in Milford, Massachusetts. The ultimate goal with LEI, a carbon dioxide laser manufacturing company, was to use an available laser, while a 1000 W laser was built that could also be synchronized to fire in a pulse of 50 milliseconds or less on the R-wave of the EKG. The available laser had an output of 320 W. The feasibility study began on patients with severe angina that had proved refractory to maximal medical care. The first patient was an 82 year old gentleman, who had previously undergone bypass graft surgery. However, this surgery had failed to relieve his severe, unrelenting angina and he was an unsuitable candidate for any other procedure. In January 1990, he consented to be the first patient to undergo TMR as a sole therapy. His pre-operative thallium scan revealed ischemic areas in the lateral and posterior walls of the left ventricle. Twenty transmural channels were placed in the appropriate regions. That the channels had passed through the entire thickness of the wall was verified by bleeding from their epicardial openings. Four days after surgery, he was completely free of angina. Furthermore, the next day he was able to exercise on a treadmill for almost ten minutes to Bruce Protocol II at 95% of the predicted heart rate without any symptoms of angina. The post-operative thallium scan lacked ischemic defects and appeared normal when examined six moths later. An additional scan performed five years after treatment also appeared normal.

CLINICAL RESULTS

The first eight TMR cases at Seton Medical Center were performed using the 320 Watt prototype laser. In these cases, we had a 50% success rate (defined as a two class reduction in angina). As mentioned, successful channel penetration to the ventricular cavity was confirmed by bleeding. The subjectivity of this method was highlighted during the operation on our sixth patient. In this case, we used transesophageal echo (TEE) to document channel penetration. The vaporization of myocardium and also blood when the laser beam passed into the ventricular cavity resulted in the formation of bubbles, which were readily visible with TEE. In fact, this method of confirming successful channel-making is now employed routinely for all TMR procedures using a carbon dioxide laser. The success ratio of channel completion with the original laser prototype was only 30%. This low value was primarily because of insufficient power; however, the presence of epicardial fat (which strongly absorbs the infrared energy), wall thickness and its effective increase if the beam was not normal to the surface, and also inadequate synchronization of the pulse to the EKG all contributed. We therefore requested that LEI design and build the 1000W carbon dioxide laser that is now used throughout the world.

The new laser used RF instead of DC stimulation and also possessed a much more sophisticated computer interface control. We used this model on our ninth patient and were able to obtain a pulse of 42 Joules with a width of 50 milliseconds. This increased power increased the channel completion rate to 90%. The failures were usually for technical reasons including the presence of epicardial fat, angulation and improper direction of the pulse.

The rest of the first fifteen patient FDA-approved feasibility study was much more successful with the new laser. We found the same positive changes in angina class, reduction in the amount of medications taken, improved exercise tolerance, and improvement of persantine thallium tests. In addition, there were no deaths or any major complications during this study (Figures 1-4).

The question of "where do the bubbles go?" was answered in part by utilization of transcranial Doppler on patient #26. The 2 MHZ probe detected bubbles at a non-significant level in the middle cerebral arterial system two to three systolic cycles after successful TMR. Computer analysis revealed that the bubble density level was insufficient to be symptomatic.

A Phase II clinical trial was then begun involving an expanded number of eight test sites. The results of this multicenter, two hundred patient, 1560 month study were reported by Horvath et al. The inclusion criteria for patients in the study were;

- intolerable angina on maximum antianginal therapy

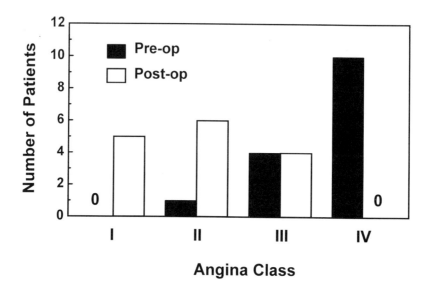

Figure 1. There was an improvement in the patients' angina class after TMR.

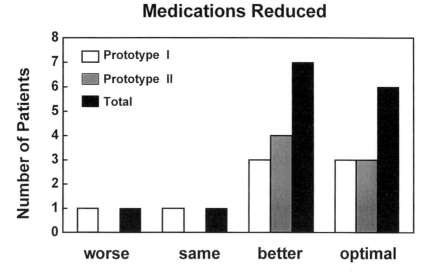

Figure 2. The patients' medications were reduced after treatment with both of the prototype carbon dioxide lasers.

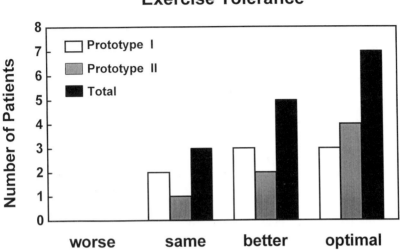

Figure 3. The majority of patients experienced an improvement in exercise tolerance after TMR.

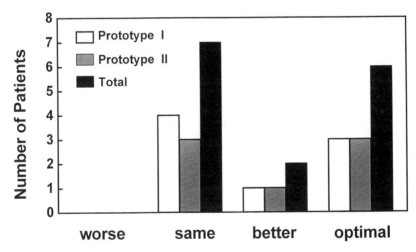

Figure 4. Thallium scans were either unchanged or improved after TMR.

- inoperability for CABG or PTCA
- evidence of ischemic targets by thallium scans

A notable favorable result of this study was a two class improvement in angina found in 75% of the patients. There was also a decreased hospitalization index from 2.5 ± 2 to 0.4 ± 0.6, and a 56% decrease in cardioactive medications. The nuclear scans revealed a decrease in ischemic defects and, in one institution, PET scans before and after the procedure confirmed improved subendocardial resting perfusion. During this study, we also discovered other parameters that influenced outcome;

- ejection fraction greater than 25% at most centers
- an overall reasonable operative risk was required (without recent myocardial infarction or acute admission into the CCU)

This became the final algorithm which was adjusted along the way by evaluating the outcomes. Acute MI, cardiac failure, low ejection fraction, and acute ischemic cardiomyopathy increased the morbidity and mortality significantly. TMR seemed not to provide a reasonable treatment for acute myocardial infarction in spite of the evidence from some of the experimental studies of acute ischemia in animal models. Other factors that we found to be important include; the number of channels (with evidence of acutely decreased compliance with too many channels), the danger of transecting the chordae tendineae with subsequent mitral valve insufficiency, or a traumatic effect with some evidence of thermal damage. Modifications of the procedure included intraoperative diuretics (given by one investigator) to counteract fluid retention in a decreasingly compliant heart and perhaps the treatment of superoxide radicals. Anticoagulants were used in varying amounts in hopes of maintaining channel patency beginning with heparin, then coumadin and almost always aspirin. Also, initially complete monitoring with Swan-Ganz, arterial line, CVP, and double lumen endotracheal intubation changed in our experience to a simple arterial line, CVP, and single lumen intubation. We have had no perioperative mortality. There have been four deaths between three and forty months, which included three cardiac events together with one brainstem stroke.

Attempts to treat the septum for anteroseptal ischemia were also performed knowing that the laser energy was dissipated in blood. The septal approach requires the ability to compress the right ventricle free of most of its blood using a large mouth probe, which prevents arrhythmias. We could then shoot directly through the wall of the right ventricle and the intraventricular septum into the left ventricular cavity. Success was again indicated by the observation of bubbles within the left ventricular chamber.

ONGOING RESEARCH

During the time of the clinical trials, several research models were used to examine the possible mechanisms of TMR. Ischemic models designed to imitate the clinical situation were tested using infarct size, survival, blood flow measurements with microspheres as end-points.

In addition, other mechanisms were proposed to explain the benefits of TMR including growth factor stimulation of collaterals, damage to sympathetic nerves, and focal thermal damage stimulating a cellular inflammatory response which indirectly stimulates intrinsic growth factor production. Several experimental studies have been designed to evaluate these possibilities. However, the basic question still remains. Where does the new blood supply come from if the intrinsic coronary artery supply is inadequate and cannot be modified? Does the growth factor stimulus create better dynamics per cell or more efficient flow with less resistance?

Corrosion Casting
We explored the basic mechanisms of TMR in a pilot study of laser-treated rabbit hearts; "Vascular corrosion casting study of TMR in rabbits". For this study, we went to Minneapolis to work with Dr. David Knighton and associates. This study used non-ischemic rabbit hearts with three channels created by the carbon dioxide laser. Hearts were excised and examined acutely and at weekly intervals up to four months after surgery. The ventricle was injected with Mercox, a synthetic resin activated to harden with a rubber-like consistency. The tissue was then dissolved with concentrated solutions of sodium and potassium hydroxide to reveal a cast of the ventricular chamber and its vascular connections. The coronary anatomy along with collaterals was examined with this technique. The finding of initial occlusion of the channels for twenty-eight days seemed to be followed by reestablishment of patency with the formation of some collateral connections (Figure 5). Histological evidence of some thermal damage with channel occlusion was evident after completion of the study probably because of excess power (35 J at 35 ms) and poor synchronization in very small and tachycardic hearts. The overall findings were

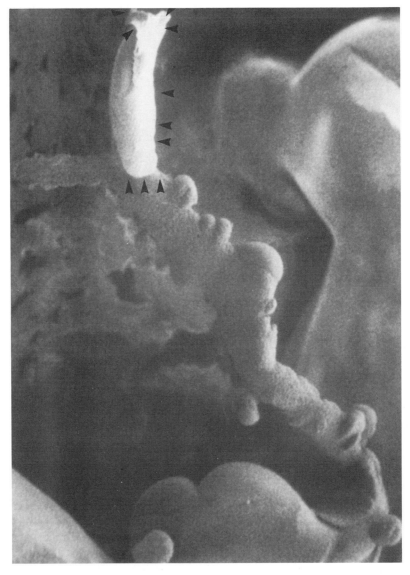

Figure 5. Corrosion cast taken from a rabbit heart twenty-eight days after channels were made with a carbon dioxide laser. An open channel connected directly to the left ventricular cavity and with apparent vascular branches is marked by the arrowheads.

inconclusive because of the above and other factors such as a non-ischemic model, competitive flow with coronary dominance due to diastolic blood flow, lack of control or assessment of coagulation factors and the intrinsic disparity of comparing the animal model to the human patient. Nevertheless, we believe that the technique has merit and in one of the specimens, a channel was demonstrated with the reestablishment of patency at twenty-eight days, which appeared to have vascular connections branching from it.

One of our patients who underwent successful TMR and who experienced a significant improvement in angina class (a reduction of three classes) with no pain on exercising or hiking, died six months after surgery because of a brainstem stroke. The patient's's heart was initially washed in saline and then fixed with a 10% formalin solution using a Foley catheter through the aortic valve as a pressure conduit with an intact mitral valve. The heart was then sent to Dr, Knighton. When infused with Mercox through the aortic valve in this closed system, blood emerged from the TMR channels. The corrosion was very difficult because of the cross-linking by formalin fixation prior to Mercox infusion. Nevertheless, the study revealed patent channels connecting to the sinusoidal or Thebesian system (Figure 6) with flow traveling out into the coronary venous confluence with apparent successful perfusion. This observation provided the first evidence of channel patency aside from the histologic studies.

Contrast Echocardiography
A new technique that clinically demonstrates TMR channel patency has been developed by investigators at the Max Planck institute in Bad Nauheim, Germany and the Schachen Clinic in Aarau, Switzerland. In a report presented at the German Society of Cardiologists in Mannheim on April 13, 1996, Dr. Klaus Berwing described the technique that allowed his group to reproducibly document perfusion taking place in the channels from the left ventricle into the myocardium. Myocardial contrast echocardiography (MCE) confirmed the presence of the contrast agent, which lasted for an average of ten heartbeats in a total of five channels around the apex of the two hearts evaluated. The contrast eventually washed out through the native vessels. However, contrast injected into bypass grafts or native coronaries could not be seen flowing in the opposite direction into the laser channels.

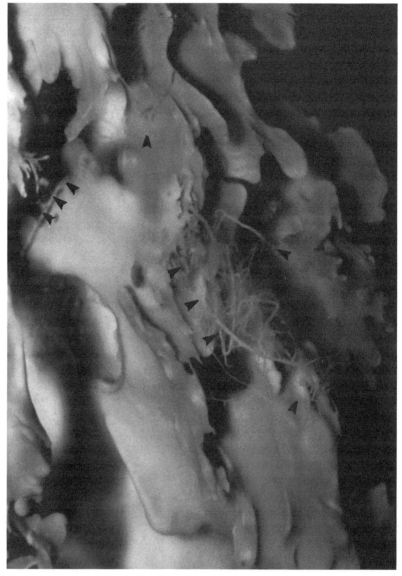

Figure 6. Corrosion cast obtained from a patient six months after TMR. The solid mass is the ventricular cavity and the vessels marked by the arrowheads represent direct connections to the cavity.

DISCUSSION

The concept of actual functional perfusion of the myocardium by these channels id difficult to understand. The first systematic attempts to map out the working of the sinusoidal network began with Wearn at the Laboratory of Experimental Medicine, Case Western Reserve University in Cleveland. He described the "myocardial sinusoids" as intermediary from the arteriole systems and that they occasionally connected into the lumen of the ventricle. Also the network of this connecting system of vascular supply to the muscle is the foundation of this TMR study, which begins with the concept of attempting to perfuse muscle with an apparent intramuscular gradient over the intracavitary ventricular end diastolic pressure. The direct nourishment of myocardial muscle fibers by blood flow differs functionally from peripheral perfusion in that myocardial blood flow occurs primarily during diastole. Systolic contraction purges the blood from the massive intravascular interconnected Thebesian network with a very quick systolic shortening of the muscle fibers. This increases intramyocardial pressure far above systolic pressure, ejecting blood into the coronary sinus. This interconnective network is very useful in cardiac surgery when coronary sinus perfusion is indicated for myocardial protection and the perfusate immediately appears in the coronary artery system. During diastole, immediate relaxation relieves the damming effect of coronary artery inflow and the muscle is briefly perfused at mostly diastolic pressures created by the closed aortic valve and peripheral resistance. At this point, the negative pressure effect within the Thebesian system created by rapid muscular fiber relaxation physically demands perfusion. This accelerated perfusion is necessary for the limited exposure time between contractions augmented by the channel per muscle flow ratio. The reptilian model of this alternate nutrient source with channels into the Thebesian system can be demonstrated histologically. The clinical correlate would be to create this type of functional channel supply with a carbon dioxide laser. The quantity of channels necessary is not known, nor is the amount of flow through these channels.

Alternative channel creation methods include other laser sources such as the holmium:YAG laser. However, in contrast to the carbon dioxide laser's high energy and long depth of focus with a single 40 ms pulse, the holmium laser delivers lower energy and requires multiple firings to complete a single channel through a fiber left inside the myocardium during several systolic contractions. Holmium is ten times less absorptive in water and with its extremely short pulse width, it essentially explodes its way through tissue by sending off an acoustic shock wave on all sides. According to Dr. Rudko of PLC, this non-vented delivery system ends up driving superheated steam into the surrounding myocardium. Histology studies indicate that the holmium leaves a wake of thermal charring and destruction of the surrounding tissue. Proponents of this method rely on the concept of the traumatic stimulation of collateral development by natural inflammatory growth factor mechanisms to explain any benefit seen.

SUMMARY

The evidence for functional channels producing at least some significant beneficial blood supply to anoxic myocardium exists. Certainly the acute clinical results, the PET scan and MCE data along with the Mercox corrosion study all point to acute benefits not possible through the collateral stimulating mechanisms described above. The areas where additional research is needed are documentation of channel blood flow along with assessment of blood flow volume, examination of the mechanism of channel reendothelialization and long-term patency, the reasons for failure of channel perfusion in some cases (which may only be temporary), and also consideration of documentable mechanisms to increase collateralization.

9

INITIAL CLINICAL EXPERIENCE WITH A HOLMIUM:YAG LASER:
A Case Study Demonstrating Increased Myocardial Perfusion

Daniel Burkhoff, Takushi Kohmoto,
Carolyn DeRosa, Craig R. Smith

Departments of Medicine and Surgery, Columbia University, New York.

INTRODUCTION

Transmyocardial laser revascularization (TMLR) has been used in many patients to effectively treat angina that is refractory to medical therapy and which cannot be treated by traditional revascularization techniques. To date, a majority of these procedures have been performed with a carbon dioxide laser. However, because of the potentially large number of patients who could benefit from such a therapy, either as sole therapy or as an adjunct to coronary bypass and angioplasty, several different types of laser energy sources have been developed for TMLR. At least two clinical trials are currently underway investigating the safety and efficacy of holmium:YAG lasers. Our institution has been participating in an international, multicenter study evaluating one such laser; the CardioGenesis ITMR System. As part of this study, fifteen patients have so far undergone TMLR as sole therapy in the United States with the CardioGenesis ITMR System and, as reported in other trials, there has been an immediate and clinically significant reduction in angina observed in most patients [1]. In this chapter, we summarize the rather dramatic results obtained in our first patient in this trial.

PATIENT CHARACTERISTICS

The patient was a forty-five year old man with a history of diabetes, hypertension and coronary artery disease. His cardiac history dates back to 1992 when he first presented with angina. Angiography at that time revealed multi-vessel coronary disease with distal vessel involvement which obviated the possibility of performing CABG. With persistent symptoms despite medical management, however, he did undergo percutaneous transluminal coronary angioplasty (PTCA) of both the anterior descending and circumflex coronary arteries later that same year. He experienced relief of angina for about two years. Over the year and a half prior to the current presentation, he has experienced a marked and progressive increase in angina which has caused significant limitations in his life style. The patient worked at the Salvation Army, a job which involved mild-to-moderate degrees of physical activity handling donated materials; however, because of frequent chest pains he was unable to work for several weeks prior to being seen at our institution. He experienced many episodes of chest pain at rest, but most of his discomfort occurred during low level exercise. He was therefore classified according to the Canadian Heart Association scale as having Class III angina. His medical regimen included calcium channel blockers (diltiazem 360 mg daily and amlodipine 10 mg daily), nitrates (isosorbide dinitrate 90 mg daily plus sublingual nitroglycerin 0.4 mg prn. ~ 15-20 per week), aspirin (325 mg daily), coumadin (10 mg daily specifically for angina), lasix (20-40 mg prn) in addition to insulin. A repeat catheterization in March of 1996 revealed the following: 50% narrowing in the mid-portion of the LAD with 90% narrowing near the apex; total occlusion of two diagonal branches with diffuse disease; total occlusion of the circumflex involving only the marginal branch which itself was diffusely diseased; total occlusion of the right coronary artery with diffuse disease of the posterior descending artery. The ejection fraction was approximately 50% with postero-basal akinesis and anterolateral and inferior hypokineses.

PREOPERATIVE ASSESSMENT AND SURGERY

Because of the diffuse nature of the disease and distal vessel involvement, neither CABG nor PTCA were considered as treatment options for this patient. Accordingly, he was offered the opportunity to participate in the IRB approved investigation studying the safety and potential efficacy of TMR with the CardioGenesis ITMR System. After an explanation of the study design and of the potential risks and benefits, the patient consented to participate. He underwent a Persantine thallium stress test during which he exhibited ischemic ECG changes (leads V_2-V_6), reversible defects in the anterior and lateral walls and a fixed posterior defect. Representative vertical long-axis views of these preoperative scans (Figure 1A) reveal the anterior defect (scans immediately after Persantine infusion are shown on the right-hand side of the figure, while corresponding rest images are shown on the left-hand side). An exercise tolerance test was performed on which he exercised to a peak heart rate of 130 beats per minute after a total of seven minutes and thirty-four seconds of the modified Bruce protocol; he experienced his typical chest pain after four minutes and forty seconds of exercise and met the ECG criteria for ischemia. Because the patient was on maximal tolerable medications, was deemed to be untreatable by other modalities and had objective evidence of ischemia, he met all of the inclusion criteria for the study. He underwent TMR in mid-April 1996 at which time twenty-two channels were created over the anterolateral wall extending from the LAD across the diagonal and obtuse marginal territories. Transesophageal echocardiography confirmed that twenty-one of the channels penetrated into the left ventricular chamber.

FOLLOW-UP

Except for a mild sized left pleural effusion, the postoperative period was uneventful and he was discharged home on the sixth postoperative day. The patient experienced significant relief of angina from the time of discharge. He gradually increased his level of activity and by eight weeks after surgery was able to resume work and enjoy daily walks and bicycle riding. At his three month follow-up visit, the patient reported marked improvement in quality of life as evidenced by his return to work, increased exercise capacity, and total elimination of sublingual nitroglycerine use. He reported experiencing angina on only two occasions; once during what he considered to be vigorous bicycle riding and once during the up-hill portion of a five mile walk. On a repeat exercise test he was able to complete ten minutes of the modified Bruce protocol to a peak heart rate of 144 beats per minute. He did experience chest pain starting at eight minutes of exercise, stopped

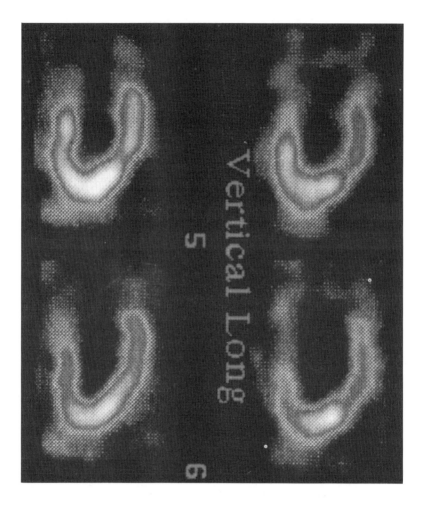

Figure 1 A. Representative preoperative vertical long-axis thallium scans obtained immediately following Persantine infusion (right side) and four hours later during rest (left side). These scans reveal the reversible anterior perfusion defect and fixed posterior defect.

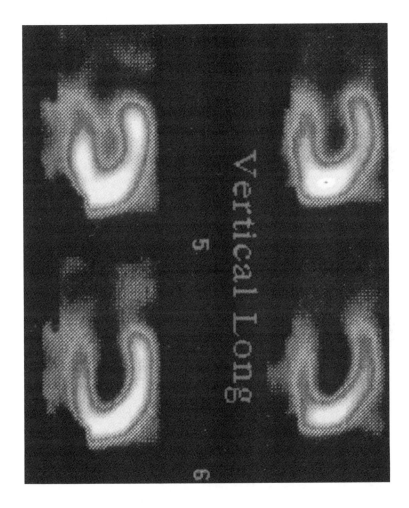

Figure 1B. Comparable scans, obtained three months after TMLR with the CardioGenesis ITMR System, again revealed the fixed posterior defect but the size and severity of the anterior defect was significantly decreased.

exercising because of shortness of breath and chest pain, but the ECG changes did not meet the criteria for ischemia. A repeat Persantine thallium test was also performed; while there was still a reversible defect in the lateral wall, the previously present anterior defect was essentially gone; vertical long-axis views of these postoperative scans are shown in Figure 1B. Also, in contrast to the preoperative test, the ECG changes during Persantine infusion did not meet the criteria for ischemia. His level of activity has continued to increase over the past month since his last follow-up visit.

DISCUSSION

As has been reported for carbon dioxide laser treatment, preliminary reports of short-term follow-up indicate that TMLR performed with the CardioGenesis ITMR System (which is built around a holmium:YAG laser) provides a reduction in angina. In this chapter, we summarize observations obtained in our first patient treated with this system. Despite prior constant medical therapy, this patient experienced a marked reduction in angina and a significant increase in exercise tolerance after laser treatment. In addition, there was objective evidence of significantly improved myocardial perfusion obtained from Persantine thallium scans. While these results are dramatic, and therefore not expected to be representative of average results obtained from a large group of patients, they do indicate that significant subjective and objective improvement in patient status can be achieved through TMLR using the CardioGenesis ITMR System. These results are reminiscent of the dramatic improvements reported anecdotally using The Heart Laser (PLC Systems, Inc.); a carbon dioxide laser.

As debate over the mechanism of action rages, results of clinical studies with different lasers (both published and unpublished reports) continue to suggest that TMLR provides a persistent reduction of angina and, in some instances improvement in myocardial flow [2-4], in otherwise untreatable patients. Although important for optimizing techniques to achieve maximum clinical benefit and for gaining widespread acceptance in the clinical community, understanding the mechanism of action is not a requirement for the thorough evaluation and clinical application of this technique which appears to be providing significant clinical benefit to suffering patients. Several long-term safety/efficacy trials are underway with different types of lasers. Different lasers may vary in some aspects of how they affect myocardial tissue, and some investigators have argued that the type of laser used is important with regard to clinical effects. Accordingly, we anticipate that significant insights into mechanisms of action will be provided by clinical results observed with these different lasers. At this early stage, results from our institution and others [1], significant clinical improvement in angina following TMLR with the CardioGenesis System has been observed.

Acknowledgment
This work was supported by a research grant from CardioGenesis Corporation, Sunnyvale, CA.

References

1. Sundt TM, Carbone KA, Oesterle SN, Robbins RC, Smith CR, Burkhoff D, Gropler RJ, Rogers JG. The holmium:YAG laser for transmyocardial laser revascularization: initial clinical results. Circulation 1996;94 (Suppl I):I-295. (abstract)
2. Frazier OH, Cooley DA, Kadipasaoglu KA, Pehlivanoglu S, Lindenmeir M, Barasch E, Conger JL, Wilansky S, Moore WH. Myocardial revascularization with laser: preliminary findings. Circulation 1995;92 (Suppl II):II-58-II-65.
3. Cooley DA, Frazier OH, Kadipasaoglu KA, Lindenmeir MH, Pehlivanoglu S, Kolff JW, Wilansky S, Moore WH. Transmyocardial laser revascularization: clinical experience with twelve-month follow-up. J Thorac Cardiovasc Surg 1996;111:791-799.
4. Horvath KA, Mannting F, Cummings N, Shernan SK, Cohn LH. Transmyocardial laser revascularization: operative techniques and clinical results at two years. J Thorac Cardiovasc Surg 1996:111:1047-1053.

10

NUCLEAR IMAGING TECHNIQUES FOR THE EVALUATION OF TMLR

Heiko Schöder, Heinrich R. Schelbert

*Division of Nuclear Medicine, Department of Molecular and Medical Pharmacology,
UCLA School of Medicine and Laboratory of Structural Biology & Molecular
Medicine*, University of California, Los Angeles, California 90095*

INTRODUCTION

Transmyocardial laser revascularization (TMLR) is currently under investigation as a novel means for augmenting regional myocardial blood flow in coronary artery disease patients unsuitable for percutaneous transluminal angioplasty (PTCA) or coronary artery bypass grafting (CABG). The laser created channels are thought to carry blood directly from the left ventricular chamber into the myocardium. Alternatively, the laser intervention may lead to an inflammatory response in the myocardium that might result in neo-angiogenesis. The clinical success of TMLR is contingent upon the net amount of additional blood flow to the ischemic myocardium and the long-term patency of the laser channels.

Radionuclide approaches appear to be particularly useful for testing the efficacy of TMLR. First, these approaches are noninvasive and thus can be readily repeated in the same patient. Second, radionuclide tracers of myocardial perfusion delineate true nutrient rather than only coronary vascular blood flow. Third, inadequate supply of blood either chronically at rest or only during exercise leads to distinct metabolic abnormalities that can be identified with radionuclide techniques. Thus, biochemical consequences of inadequate blood flow as well as metabolic responses to TMLR can be demonstrated with radiotracers of myocardial substrate metabolism. Lastly, radionuclide approaches also permit the simultaneous assessment of ventricular function and myocardial perfusion.

RADIONUCLIDE IMAGING OF MYOCARDIAL BLOOD FLOW AND METABOLISM

Imaging Instrumentation

Two conceptually different imaging modalities are available; (a) the widely available single photon emission computed tomography (SPECT) and, (b) the more sophisticated Positron Emission Tomography (PET). Table 1 summarizes the major differences between both imaging approaches. These differences depend largely on the radioactive elements and their physical decay characteristics. Both modalities yield images of high diagnostic quality. SPECT offers an intrinsic spatial resolution of about 10 to 12 mm that depends also on the distance between the object imaged and the photon detecting device. Further, its relatively low temporal resolution precludes measurements of rapidly changing tracer tissue activity concentrations as for example in blood and myocardium. SPECT therefore assesses primarily the relative distribution of radiotracers in the left ventricular myocardium and, thus, yields qualitative information on regional myocardial tissue function. In addition to myocardial blood flow, regional myocardial metabolism can also be evaluated, at least to some extent, with radioiodinated fatty acid analogs (Table 2).

In contrast, PET offers a broad spectrum of radiotracers that allow an assessment of not only myocardial blood flow, but also of various aspects of the myocardial substrate metabolism as well as neuronal activity and function (as illustrated in Table 2).

Table 1. Comparison of Single Photon and Positron Emission Tomography Imaging

	SPECT	PET
Physical principle	single photon emission radiation	coincidence detection of annihilation radiation caused by positron decay
Collimation	lead collimation	electron collimation
Spatial resolution	10-12 mm	3-4 mm
Attenuation correction	optional	routine
Quantification	no	yes
Availability	+++	+ (+)

Table 2. Radiotracers and -pharmaceuticals used for SPECT and PET imaging

Technique	Tracer	Parameter studied
SPECT	Tc99m sestamibi	myocardial perfusion
	Tc99m tetrofosmin	
	Tl-201 chloride	myocardial perfusion
	I-123 BMIPP	fatty acid uptake
	I-123 MIBG	sympathetic innervation
PET	O-15 water*	myocardial blood flow
	N-13 ammonia*	
	Rb-82	
	Cu-62 PTSM	
	F-18 deoxyglucose	glucose utilization
	C-11 palmitate	fatty acid oxidation
	C-11 acetate	oxidative metabolism (myocardial blood flow*)
	C-11 hydroxyephedrine	sympathetic innervation

(*for further explanation see text)

This is because positron emitting isotopes of elements like carbon, nitrogen, oxygen and fluorine all abundantly present in nature, can be inserted into biochemically active compounds without modifying their biologic properties. Besides the high depth-independent spatial resolution that approaches 4 to 5 mm, PET images are corrected for photon attenuation so that they reflect quantitatively regional myocardial tracer activity concentrations. Temporal resolution rates ranging from one to several seconds allow measurements of rapid changes in tracer tissue concentrations so that several functional processes (as for example myocardial blood flow, oxygen consumption and glucose utilization) can be measured in absolute units of mL blood or mmol substrates/min/g myocardium.

Assessment of Myocardial Blood Flow
Regional myocardial blood flow as one of the important parameters in the evaluation of patients before and after TMLR can be evaluated qualitatively with SPECT with either Tl-201 or Tc-99m labeled sestamibi or tetrofosmin. Several tracers of blood flow including O-15 water, Rubidium-82 and N-13 ammonia are available with PET. Besides semiquantitative assessments of the relative distribution of myocardial blood flow estimates of absolute blood flow in mL/min/g myocardium can be obtained with O-15 water, N-13 ammonia and as demonstrated more recently, with Rubidium-82 [1-6].

Assessment of Myocardial Substrate Metabolism
For the assessment and quantification of regional myocardial oxidative metabolism or oxygen consumption, either C-11 acetate [7-10] or molecular O-15 oxygen [11, 12] are available. The uptake of free fatty acid as the myocardium's preferred fuel substrate and its relative distribution between immediate oxidation (including beta-oxidation and tricarboxylic acid cycle activity) and initial deposition of free fatty acid into the endogenous lipid pools can be evaluated with C-11 palmitate [13, 14]. More recently, absolute measurements of fatty acid oxidation have become available with this tracer [15]. Further, regional myocardial utilization rates of glucose can be evaluated or even be measured in absolute unites with the glucose analog, F-18 2-fluoro-2-deoxyglucose (FDG) [16, 17]. The tracer exchanges across the capillary and cell membranes in proportion to glucose; it then competes with glucose for hexokinase to be phosphorylated to FDG-6-phosphate. The phosphorylated metabolite becomes virtually trapped in the myocardium so that regional F-18 activity concentrations reflect regional rates of exogenous glucose utilization.

RADIONUCLIDE STUDIES IN PATIENTS AFTER TMLR

Clinical Indications
The generally accepted inclusion criteria for TMLR are; (a) severe angina pectoris refractory to medical treatment, (b) reversible ischemia as demonstrated by myocardial perfusion imaging, and (c) target vessels unsuitable for interventional revascularization.

Clinically relevant questions that radionuclide techniques can answer prior to TMLR include the following;

- Does the patient have reversible regional myocardial dysfunction at rest?
- Does stress, either physical or pharmacologically induced, cause regional myocardial perfusion defects?
- If so, what are the metabolic consequences of either rest or stress-induced perfusion defects?

Following TMLR an improvement in anginal status and overall symptoms and well being have been reported [18-21]. However, because these parameters are highly subjective they require objective verification. Radionuclide techniques can answer several clinically relevant questions following treatment;

- Has regional nutrient myocardial blood flow increased at rest and/or during stress?
- Have metabolic consequences of inadequate blood flow resolved or improved?
- Does the improvement in perfusion and/or metabolism correlate with improvements in regional wall motion, symptoms and exercise capacity?
- If so, do these improvements persist over prolonged time periods?
- Has TMLR itself resulted in scar tissue formation?

Assessment of Myocardial Perfusion and Left Ventricular Function
Myocardial perfusion imaging can be used to verify reversible ischemia as one of the major inclusion criteria and an improvement in resting and exercise perfusion following TMLR. Myocardial blood flow can be quantified by three approaches;

- as absolute myocardial blood flow (MBF), only measurable with PET and

expressed as mL/min/g tissue;
- by comparing interregional differences within the myocardium, and
- as myocardial flow reserve, that is the ratio of blood flow during exercise or pharmacologically induced stress over blood flow at rest.

For clinical routine, images are resliced into short and long axis cuts of the left ventricle and perfusion defects classified according to their location, extent, severity and reversibility. These perfusion defects primarily indicate a disparity of blood flow distribution within the myocardium and not necessarily myocardial ischemia. For instance, perfusion defects at rest may indicate myocardial infarction, resting ischemia or hibernating myocardium. Likewise, new perfusion defects during exercise imaging reflect areas with reduced flow reserve, i.e. less increase in blood flow compared to normally perfused myocardium (a real decline in absolute blood flow, refereed to as "stealing", occurs rarely in the clinical setting). Finally, new perfusion defects following TMLR could indicate the presence of scar tissue formed as direct result of laser-mediated thermal injury.

Initial Observations with Radionuclide Techniques in TMLR Patients
Several investigations have employed the advantages of radionuclide approaches for assessing the efficacy of TMLR. Controversy exists whether laser channels can provide an *immediate* benefit to ischemic myocardium; more likely, these channels may, *over time*, have a protective effect [22-27]. Indeed, some preliminary clinical studies show such improvement in myocardial perfusion over time [18, 20, 28-30].

In a multicenter study, Horvath et al [30] followed two hundred patients treated with TMLR over a time of 10 ± 3 months. All patients underwent stress/rest SPECT imaging with either Tl-201 or Tc-99m sestamibi prior to operation. The radionuclide studies were repeated on follow-up at three and six months, while follow-up at twelve months was available in only 50% of patients. As shown in Figure 1 the number of exercise induced, reversible perfusion defects was significantly decreased at three months and continued to decline over the subsequent follow-up period.

Of note, no such improvement in myocardial perfusion was found in a subset of patients at one of the participating centers of this multicenter study [20,29]. On follow-up at three and twelve months there was no change in myocardial perfusion assessed by Tl-201 SPECT. One year after TMLR, the relative blood flow to laser treated segments was $51\pm23\%$ of that found in the normal territories as compared

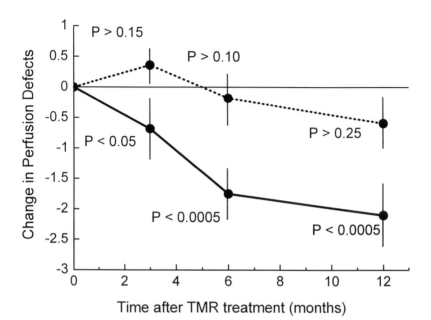

Figure 1. Changes in myocardial perfusion defects after TMLR. The solid line represents reversible perfusion defects and the dashed line fixed defects. The number of reversible perfusion defects, indicating stress-induced myocardial ischemia, decreased significantly after laser treatment while no increase in fixed perfusion defects, indicative of perioperative or subsequent myocardial infarction, was observed. Follow-up after two, six, and twelve months was performed in 120, 107, and 59 patients respectively. (Reprinted with permission from J Thorac Cardiovasc Surg [ref 30], Mosby Year Book).

to $45 \pm 21\%$ at baseline. While these data suggest a 13% increase in relative regional blood flow, the increase failed to achieve statistical significance.

The unique features of PET, i.e. the ability to quantify myocardial blood flow, have not been used yet to study the effects of TMLR. A semiquantitative approach was chosen by Frazier et al who studied twenty-one patients prior to and following laser revascularization using N-13 ammonia and PET imaging [20]. Based on the assumption that laser channels may occlude towards the epicardial surface of the heart, but their subendocardial portion remains patent, they derived a subendo- to subepicardial perfusion ratio. This ratio increased from 0.88 ± 0.03 prior to TMLR to 1.05 ± 0.04 at three months and 1.11 ± 0.02 at six months of follow-up. Similar data were reported in a subset of these patients with up to twelve months of follow-up [29]. These interesting findings appear to explain the improvement in functional class and exercise tolerance that was also reported [20]. However, the methodological approach used in these studies has limitations. Given the spatial resolution of even the newest generation of PET scanners, a true increase in subendocardial blood flow is unlikely to be measurable, in particular when PET studies are not gated. The authors acknowledge these limitations, but claim that their approach shows at least qualitative directional trends in the subendo- to subepicardial perfusion ratio [20]. Of note, no changes in regional perfusion were found when the total transmural blood flow was assessed in laser treated left ventricular myocardium.

Potential Applications of Radionuclide Techniques in TMLR Patients
Although these initial observations seem to support the utility of TMLR, they do not necessarily answer the question of whether tissue blood flow has indeed been restored adequately. One approach to answering this question is an assessment of regional myocardial wall motion at rest or, if normal, during pharmacological or physical stress. Several radiotracers are available for the evaluation of regional and global left ventricular function. Gated image acquisition with Tc-99m labeled perfusion agents permits the *simultaneous* assessment of myocardial perfusion and contractile function [31, 32]. Functional parameters that can be assessed include regional and global ejection fraction, as well as regions of asynchronous contraction. Theoretically gated FDG imaging also allows evaluation of left ventricular wall motion and ejection fraction. However, this method is not used routinely at the present time.

A second approach, especially in instances of large regions that have been revascularized, include *quantitative* measurements of myocardial blood flow. Blood flow largely depends on myocardial oxygen consumption, which in turn is governed by cardiac work. Numerous studies have established statistically significant direct correlations between measurements of myocardial blood flow and the rate pressure product as a readily available index of cardiac work [33, 34]. Thus, regional myocardial blood flow, normalized for the actual cardiac work, can indicate the adequacy of revascularization. As another possibility, the response of regional myocardial blood flow to either pharmacological or physical stress can be determined. Absence of stress induced defects as assessed qualitatively with either SPECT or more quantitatively with PET would support the claim that TMLR has indeed been adequate.

There may be limitations, however, to the use of pharmacologically induced hyperemia employing either intravenous dipyridamole or adenosine. Both agents exert their profound vasodilator effect by direct vascular smooth muscle relaxation. If TMLR has not resulted in angiogenesis, then neither agent seems likely to increase flow through the laser created channels. In this situation, true increases in myocardial oxygen demand by physical stress or by inotropic stimulation (with, for example, dobutamine or arbutamine) would result in a local release of metabolites causing an increase in myocardial blood flow and thus more likely demonstrate the efficacy of laser channels.

Possibilities for Identifying Metabolic Consequences of Ischemia and Potential Reversibility of Contractile Dysfunction
The metabolic consequences of myocardial ischemia can be assessed with a number of radiotracers. Thus, acute stress induced ischemia is known to be associated with reductions in oxidative metabolism and in fatty acid oxidation, which can be detected with either C-11 acetate or C-11 palmitate acetate [7-10, 13, 14, 35]. While their initial uptake into the myocardium depends largely on myocardial blood flow, the subsequent clearance from the myocardium correlates in the case of C-11 acetate with flux through the TCA cycle or, in the case of C-11 palmitate, with the rate of myocardial beta-oxidation *and* flux through the TCA cycle. From a purely technical point of view, the regional tracer tissue clearance rate, as determined from serially acquired images, yields, in conjunction with the initial tracer uptake, a more robust and more easily detectable signal than the clearance rate alone. Impairments of fatty acid metabolism would be reflected on the biexponential tissue clearance curve by a decrease in the fraction of the fatty acid tracer that immediately enters oxidation, as well as a decrease in its rate of clearance from the myocardium. Conversely, improvements in fatty acid oxidation would be reflected by corresponding changes in the tissue clearance curve morphology. For instance, the relative size of the rapid clearance phase as a reflection of the tracer amount that becomes immediately oxidized would increase together with an acceleration of the tracer clearance from the myocardium. Similar changes would be observed with C-11 acetate. As the tissue clearance rate

correlates with the flux through the TCA cycle, ischemia would be associated with a diminished clearance rate while a post-revascularization improvement in oxidative metabolism would be associated with higher clearance rates. Similar patterns and changes are likely to be noted in dysfunctional myocardium at rest.

Myocardial ischemia also produces a marked increase in glucose utilization together with an impairment in fatty acid utilization and oxidative metabolism, i.e. TCA cycle flux. Associated with increased lactate release, the enhanced glucose uptake reflects increased anaerobic glycolysis. This regional shift in substrate usage has been demonstrated in animal experiments as well as in patients with coronary artery disease, either during or immediately after exercise testing. However, it is also observed frequently in dysfunctional myocardium in patients with chronic coronary artery disease, but *without* clinical evidence of acute myocardial ischemia. It remains uncertain, whether the mechanisms accounting for the augmentation of regional glucose uptake during *acute* ischemia can be extrapolated to the situation of *chronic* myocardial contractile dysfunction. Nevertheless, the persistence of enhanced FDG uptake in hypoperfused and dysfunctional myocardium has been established as a marker of "myocardial viability". Evidence suggests that this phenomenon is related to a change in the expression of membrane glucose transporters [36, 37].

The term "myocardial viability" is frequently used to describe reversibility of left ventricular dysfunction. The assessment of reversible contractile dysfunction is of importance in patients with multivessel coronary artery disease and reduced left ventricular function and those in whom coronary revascularization is considered a treatment option but perfusion imaging does not clearly detect areas of reversible ischemia. [38-41]. The presence and extent of viable myocardium are closely related to the post-revascularization improvement in left ventricular function [42-48], an improvement in heart failure symptoms [49] and survival [42-44]. Therefore, the detection of viable myocardium might considerably influence the treatment strategy: patients could either be treated medically, undergo coronary revascularization including TMLR or cardiac transplantation.

Typically, the assessment of such reversible contractile dysfunction entails the evaluation of regional myocardial blood flow followed by the search for persistent glucose metabolic activity in hypoperfused myocardial regions. Normal or enhanced FDG uptake in hypoperfused myocardial regions, a scenario referred to as blood flow/metabolism mismatch, signifies reversibility of contractile dysfunction. In contrast, a reduction in glucose utilization corresponding to the reduction in myocardial blood flow is referred to as blood flow/metabolism match and is associated with a low likelihood for recovery of contractile dysfunction. Such flow metabolism patterns have been demonstrated to be highly accurate in predicting the post-revascularization outcome in regional contractile function.[45, 47, 48, 50, 51].

From a technical point of view, because glucose uptake in reversibly dysfunctional myocardial regions is characteristically enhanced, it is easily recognizable on the blood flow/metabolism images. This is in contrast to other approaches for assessing the potential reversibility of regional contractile dysfunction as for example with the cation Tl-201. With thallium, the initial tracer uptake reflects regional myocardial blood flow. Over time, the tracer equilibrates with the myocardial potassium pools, so that "filling in" of defects on delayed thallium imaging indicates the presence of viable myocardium. However, subtle changes in regional thallium activity concentrations may be difficult to recognize. This is in contrast to the positive signal of FDG uptake, so that combined perfusion/glucose metabolism imaging, for instance with N-13 ammonia/FDG, is considered the gold standard for the detection of viable myocardium.

Several alternate approaches for the assessment of myocardial viability have been proposed. Their common principle is that they are based on threshold levels for either myocardial perfusion or metabolism. For instance, it has been demonstrated that reversible contractile dysfunction characteristically is associated with either normal or only modestly reduced tissue clearance rates of C-11 acetate, whereas the clearance rates were more severely reduced in irreversibly dysfunctional myocardial regions [8, 35]. In addition, the extent of residual myocardial blood flow has been noted to be correlated closely with the regional amount of myocardial fibrosis [52, 53]. Other studies based on the fraction of myocardium that rapidly exchanges water [54, 55], or on biopsy specimens obtained during coronary artery bypass grafting [52, 53, 56, 57], have established a fibrosis fraction of 35-40% as a threshold for recovery of contractile function. For example, if the amount of fibrosis in a myocardial segment exceeds 30-40%, its contractile function is unlikely to improve with revascularization. Therefore, very mild flow reductions imply little or no fibrosis as compared to very severe flow reductions that are usually associated with extensive fibrosis and, hence, irreversibility of contractile dysfunction. However, intermediate flow reductions are of limited value in predicting whether contractile function will or will not improve following revascularization.

Because TMLR may lead to only small or subtle improvements in regional flow, they may remain undetectable by either SPECT or PET blood flow imaging. Yet, even a small augmentation in flow may lessen the metabolic consequences of either resting or stress-induced hypoperfusion. Such amelioration of metabolic alterations could be tested with radionuclide techniques evaluating regional myocardial substrate metabolism. Lastly, the formation of scar tissue in response to TMLR could equally well be determined by simultaneous evaluation of regional myocardial blood flow and metabolism.

CONCLUSION

In conclusion, even though several studies have shown an improvement in functional class and relieve of angina pectoris in patients with coronary artery disease after TMLR, the morphologic background and the pathophysiological mechanisms involved still remain somewhat speculative. It is surprising that a new surgical technique whose effectiveness has not been proven convincingly, is currently applied to treat thousands of patients worldwide. Clearly, large multicenter trials are needed to establish the exact role of TMLR in the treatment of patients with coronary artery disease. It should be emphasized that the ultimate parameter to evaluate the success of TMLR is not, as is often published, freedom from angina pectoris. Although angina class might considerably affect the patients quality of life, a surgical intervention with the only gain of relieving angina pectoris would hardly be justifiable and certainly not be cost-effective. It is therefore of particular interest, that nuclear medicine imaging provides the necessary and cost-effective armamentarium to verify changes in myocardial perfusion, metabolism and function following TMLR.

Acknowledgments
The authors are grateful to Diane Martin for preparing the illustration and to Eileen Rosenfeld for her skillful secretarial assistance in preparing the manuscript.

*Operated for the U.S. Department of Energy by the University of California under Contract #DE-AC03-76-SF00012. This work was supported in part by the Director of the Office of Energy Research, Office of Health and Environmental Research, Washington D.C., by Research Grants #HL 29845 and #HL 33177, National Institutes of Health, Bethesda, MD and by an Investigative Group Award by the Greater Los Angeles Affiliate of the American Heart Association, Los Angeles, CA.

References

1. Nitzsche EU, Choi Y, Czernin J, Hoh CK, Huang SC, Schelbert HR. Noninvasive quantification of myocardial blood flow in humans. A direct comparison of the [13N]ammonia and the [15O]water techniques. Circulation 1996;93:2000-2006.
2. Araujo L, Lammertsma A, Rhodes C, et al. Noninvasive quantification of regional myocardial blood flow in coronary artery disease with oxygen-15-labeled carbon dioxide inhalation and positron emission tomography. Circulation 1991;83:875-885.
3. Bergmann SR, Herrero P, Markham J, Weinheimer CJ, Walsh MN. Noninvasive quantitation of myocardial blood flow in human subjects with oxygen-15-labeled water and positron emission tomography. J Am Coll Cardiol 1989;14:639-652.
4. Hutchins G, Schwaiger M, Rosenspire K, Krivokapich J, Schelbert H, Kuhl D. Noninvasive quantification of regional blood flow in the human heart using N-13 ammonia and dynamic positron emission tomographic imaging. J Am Coll Cardiol 1990;15:1032-1042.
5. Kuhle WG, Porenta G, Huang SC, et al. Quantification of regional myocardial blood flow using 13N-ammonia and reoriented dynamic positron emission tomographic imaging. Circulation 1992;86:1004-1017.
6. Bol A, Melin JA, Vanoverschelde JL, et al. Direct comparison of [13N]ammonia and [15O]water estimates of perfusion with quantification of regional myocardial blood flow by microspheres. Circulation 1993;87:512-525.
7. Armbrecht JJ, Buxton DB, Schelbert HR. Validation of [1-^{11}C] acetate as a tracer for noninvasive assessment of oxidative metabolism with positron emission tomography in normal, ischemic, post-ischemic and hyperemic canine myocardium. Circulation 1991;81:1594-1605.
8. Gropler RJ, Siegel BA, Sampathkumaran K, et al. Dependence of recovery of contractile function on maintenance of oxidative metabolism after myocardial infarction. J Am Coll Cardiol 1992;19:989-997.
9. Brown MA, Myears DW, Bergmann SR. Noninvasive assessment of canine myocardial oxidative metabolism with 11C-acetate and positron emission tomography. J Am Coll Cardiol 1988;12:1054-1063.
10. Brown MA, Myears DW, Bergmann SR. Validity of estimates of myocardial oxidative metabolism with carbon-11 acetate and positron emission tomography despite altered patterns of substrate utilization. J Nucl Med 1989;30:187-193.
11. Iida H, Rhodes CG, Araujo LI, et al. Noninvasive quantification of regional myocardial metabolic rate for oxygen by use of 15O2 inhalation and positron emission tomography. Theory, error analysis, and application in humans. Circulation 1996;94:792-807.
12. Yamamoto Y, de Silva R, Rhodes CG, et al. Noninvasive quantification of regional myocardial metabolic rate of oxygen by 15O2 inhalation and positron emission tomography. Experimental validation. Circulation 1996;94:808-816.
13. Schön HR, Schelbert HR, Najafi A, et al. C-11 labeled palmitic acid for the noninvasive evaluation of regional myocardial fatty acid metabolism with positron

computed tomography. I. Kinetics of C-11 palmitic acid in normal myocardium. Am Heart J 1982;103:532-547.

14. Schön H, Senekowitsch R, Berg D. Measurement of myocardial fatty acid metabolism: Kinetics of iodine-123-heptadecanoic acid in normal dog hearts. J Nucl Med 1986;27:1449.

15. Bergmann SR, Weinheimer CJ, Markham J, Herrero P. Quantitation of myocardial fatty acid metabolism using PET. J Nucl Med 1996;37:1723-1730.

16. Krivokapich J, Huang SC, Selin CE, Phelps ME, Schelbert HR. Fluorodeoxyglucose rate constants, lumped constant, and glucose metabolic rate in rabbit heart. Am J Physiol 1987;252:H777-H787.

17. Gambhir SS, Schwaiger M, Huang SC, et al. Simple noninvasive quantification method for measuring myocardial glucose utilization in humans employing positron emission tomography and Fluorine-18 deoxyglucose. J Nucl Med 1989;30:359-366.

18. Crew JR, Thuener M, Jones R, Ryan C, Chimenti C, Fisher JC. Transmyocardial laser revascularization. J Am Coll Cardiol 1994;23:151A. (abstract)

19. Donovan CL, Landolfo KP, Lowe JE, Clements F, Coleman RB, Ryan T. Improvement in inducible ischemia during dobutamine stress echocardiography after transmyocardial laser revascularization in patients with refractory angina. J Am Coll Cardiol 1997;30:607-612.

20. Frazier OH, Cooley DA, Kadipasaoglu KA, et al. Myocardial revascularization with laser. Preliminary findings. Circulation 1995;92 (suppl.II):II-58-II-65.

21. Nägele H, Kalmar P, Lübeck M, et al. Transmyokardiale Laserrevaskularisation - Behandlungsoption der koronaren Herzerkrankung? (Transmyocardial laser revascularization - treatment option for coronary artery disease?). Z Kardiol 1997;86:171-178.

22. Hardy RI, James FW, Millard RW, Kaplan S. Regional myocardial blood flow and cardiac mechanics in dogs with CO2 laser induced intramyocardial revascularization. Basic Res Cardiol 1990;85:179-197.

23. Landreneau R, Nawarawong W, Laughlin H et al. Direct CO2 laser revascularization of the myocardium. Lasers Surg Med 1991;11:35-42.

24. Goda T, Wierzbicki Z, Gaston A, Leandri J, Vouron J, Loisance D. Myocardial revascularization by CO2 laser. Eur Surg Res 1987;19:113-117.

25. Whittaker P, Kloner RA, Przyklenk K. Laser-mediated transmural channels do not salvage acutely ischemic myocardium. J Am Coll Cardiol 1993;22:302-309.

26. Gassler N, Wintzer HO, Stubbe HM, Wullbrand A, Helmchen U. Transmyocardial laser revascularization. Histological features in human nonresponder myocardium. Circulation 1997;95:371-375.

27. Schäper F, Lipper F, Krabatsch T, Blümcke S. Results of histomorphological and histomorphometrical investigations of left ventricular myocardium after transmyocardial laser revascularization. J Am Coll Cardiol 1997;29:73A. (abstract)

28. Kakavas PW, March RJ, Macioch JE, et al. Effects of transmyocardial laser revascularization on regional left ventricular function and contractile reserve: evaluation by resting and dobutamine stress echocardiography. Circulation

1995;92, Suppl I:I-176. (abstract)

29. Cooley DA, Frazier OH, Kadipasaoglu KA, Pehlivanoglu S, Shannon RL, Angelini P. Transmyocardial laser revascularization: anatomic evidence of long-term channel patency. Texas Heart Inst J 1994;21:220-224.

30. Horvath KA, Cohn LH, Cooley DA, et al. Transmyocardial laser revascularization: results of a multi-center trial with transmyocardial laser revascularization as sole therapy for end stage coronary artery disease. J Thorac Cardiovasc Surg 1997;113:645-653.

31. DePuey EG, Nichols K, Dobrinsky C. Left ventricular ejection fraction assessment from gated technetium-99m sestamibi SPECT. J Nucl Med 1993;34:1871-1876.

32. Mochizuki T, Murase K, Tanaka H, Hamamoto K, Tauxe WN. Assessment of left ventricular volume using ECG-gated SPECT with technetium-99m-MIBI and technetium-99m-tetrofosmin. J Nucl Med 1997;38:53-57.

33. Klocke FJ, Mattes RE, Lanty JM, Ellis AK. Pressure-flow relationship. Controversial issues and probable implications. Circ Res 1985;56:239-299.

34. Czernin J, Müller P, Chan S, et al. Influence of age and hemodynamics on myocardial blood flow and flow reserve. Circulation 1993;88:62-69.

35. Buxton DB, Vaghaiwalla-Mody F, Krivokapich J, Phelps ME, Schelbert HR. Quantitative assessment of prolonged metabolic abnormalities in reperfused canine myocardium. Circulation 1992;85:1842-1856.

36. Young LH, Renfu Y, Russell R, et al. Low-flow ischemia leads to translocation of canine heart GLUT-4 and GLUT-1 glucose transporters to the sarcolemma in vivo Circulation 1997;95:415-422.

37. Brosius Fr, Liu Y, Nguyen N, Sun D, Bartlett J, Schwaiger M. Persistent myocardial ischemia increases GLUT1 glucose transporter expression in both ischemic and non-ischemic heart regions. J Mol Cell Cardiol 1997;29:1675-1685.

38. Iskandrian AS, Heo J, Stanberry C. When is myocardial viability an important clinical issue? J Nucl Med 1994;35 (suppl):4S-7S.

39. Maddahi J, Schelbert H, Brunken R, Di Carli M. Role of thallium-201 and PET imaging in evaluation of myocardial viability and management of patients with coronary artery disease and left ventricular dysfunction. J Nucl Med 1994; 35:707-715.

40. Schelbert H. Positron emission tomography for the assessment of myocardial viability. Circulation 1991;84 (suppl I):I-122-I-131.

41. Schöder H, Friedrich M, Topp H. Myocardial viability: what do we need? Eur J Nucl Med 1993;20:792-803.

42. Di Carli MF, Davidson M, Little R, et al. Value of metabolic imaging with positron emission tomography for evaluating prognosis in patients with coronary artery disease and left ventricular dysfunction. Am J Cardiol 1994;73:527-533.

43. Eitzman D, Al-Aouar Z, Kanter HL, et al. Clinical outcome of patients with advanced coronary artery disease after viability studies with positron emission tomography. J Am Coll Cardiol 1992;20:559-565.

44. Lee KS, Marwick TH, Cook SA, et al. Prognosis of patients with left ventricular dysfunction, with and without viable myocardium after myocardial infarction.

Relative efficacy of medical therapy and revascularization. Circulation 1994;90:2687-2694.

45. Tillisch J, Brunken R, Marshall R, et al. Reversibility of cardiac wall motion abnormalities predicted by positron tomography. N Engl J Med 1986;314:884-888.

46. Tamaki N, Yonekura Y, Yamashita K, et al. Positron emission tomography using fluorine-18 deoxyglucose in evaluation of coronary artery bypass grafting. Am J Cardiol 1989;64:860-865.

47. Lucignani G, Paolini G, Landoni C, et al. Presurgical identification of hibernating myocardium by combined use of technetium-99m hexakis 2-methoxyisobutylisonitrile single photon emission tomography and fluorine-18 fluoro-2-deoxy-D-glucose positron emission tomography in patients with coronary artery disease. Eur J Nucl Med 1992;19:874-881.

48. Gropler RJ, Geltman EM, Sampathkumaran K, et al. Functional recovery after coronary revascularization for chronic coronary artery disease is dependent on maintenance of oxidative metabolism. J Am Coll Cardiol 1992;20:569-577.

49. Di Carli M, Asgarzadie F, Schelbert HR, et al. Quantitative relation between myocardial viability and improvement in heart failure symptoms after revascularization in patients with ischemic cardiomyopathy. Circulation 1995;92:3436-3444.

50. Tamaki N, Kawamoto M, Tadamura E, et al. Prediction of reversible ischemia after revascularization: perfusion and metabolic studies using positron emission tomography. Circulation 1995;91:1697-1705

51. Tamaki N, Ohtani H, Yamashita K, et al. Metabolic activity in the areas of new fill-in after thallium-201 reinjection: comparison with Positron Emission Tomography using fluorine-18-deoxyglucose. J Nucl Med 1991;32:673-678.

52. Deprè C, Vanoverschelde J, Melin J, et al. Structural and metabolic correlates of the reversibility of chronic left ventricular ischemic dysfunction in humans. Am J Physiol 1995;268:H1265-H1275.

53. Maes A, Flameng W, Nuyts J, et al. Histological alterations in chronically hypoperfused myocardium. Circulation 1994;90:735-745.

54. Yamamoto Y, de Silva R, Rhodes C, et al. A new strategy for the assessment of viable myocardium and regional myocardial blood flow using ^{15}O-Water and Dynamic Positron Emission Tomography. Circulation 1992;86:167-178.

55. de Silva R, Yamamoto Y, Rhodes CG, et al. Preoperative prediction of the outcome of coronary revascularization using positron emission tomography. Circulation 1992;86:1738-1742.

56. Shivalkar B, Maes A, Borgers M, et al. Only hibernating myocardium invariably shows early recovery after coronary revascularization. Circulation 1996;94:308-315.

57. Schwarz ER, Schaper J, vom Dahl J, et al. Myocyte degeneration and cell death in hibernating human myocardium. J Am Coll Cardiol 1996;27:1577-1585.

11

MYOCARDIAL ANGIOGENESIS: BIOLOGY AND THERAPY

Charles A. Mack[1,2], Shailen R. Patel[1,2], Christopher J. Magovern[1], Ronald G. Crystal,[2] Todd K. Rosengart[1]

[1]*Department of Cardiothoracic Surgery and* [2]*Division of Pulmonary and Critical Care Medicine, The New York Hospital-Cornell Medical Center, New York, New York.*

INTRODUCTION

Despite significant advances in its prevention and treatment, coronary artery disease (CAD) remains the leading cause of death in the Western world today. The economic burden of CAD on society is significant. It has been estimated that the annual cost of treating the approximately 6.3 million Americans afflicted with this disease is $56 billion, with CAD accounting for a significant proportion of the total number of work days lost to illness in the United States [1,2]. Conventional treatment for CAD includes medical therapies designed to reduce hypercholesterolemia, prevent disease progression and reduce myocardial oxygen demand; and interventional therapies that restore blood flow to the epicardial coronary vessels, either by angioplasty or bypass surgery.

The original premise for transmyocardial laser revascularization (TMR) was that myocardial perfusion could be enhanced by creating channels that would allow direct perfusion of the ischemic tissue from the left ventricular chamber [3,4]. However, recent studies have suggested that TMR may increase myocardial perfusion by stimulating angiogenesis [5-9], a biological process that mediates development of new blood vessels in the post-embryonic state. In this context, an understanding of the biology of angiogenesis is relevant to any discussion of TMR. Furthermore, recent advances in elucidating the biology of angiogenesis, including the discovery of a number of proteins that induce angiogenesis, has made possible the consideration of therapeutic enhancement of this process - a strategy known as "therapeutic angiogenesis." Therapeutic angiogenesis may be useful as an adjunctive measure in augmenting the benefits of TMR.

BIOLOGY OF ANGIOGENESIS

Development of the vasculature is essential for providing vertebrate tissues with oxygen and metabolic nutrients, and removing the products of metabolism. The process of "vasculogenesis" occurs during embryologic development, and is characterized by the *de novo* formation of new blood vessels from angioblasts, which results in the formation of large vessels [10]. Vasculogenesis occurs within yolk sac mesoderm as a condensation of undifferentiated mesenchymal cells to form angiogenic cell clusters which, in turn, form blood-forming elements and blood vessels. Later in embryologic life, the major, large blood vessels burrow into each organ and form anastomoses with capillary beds within that organ [11]. The term "angiogenesis" is usually applied when new blood vessels sprout from pre-existing vessels. Such development occurs mainly in the post-embryological period [8,9,12].

The postembryonic angiogenesis process occurs in a sequence that involves: (1) disruption of basement membranes, (2) remodeling (usually degradation) of the extracellular matrix ; (3) migration of endothelial cells; (4) and their subsequent proliferation; and finally (5) the organization of tube-like constructs of endothelial cells which eventually become the new vessels [8,9] (Figure 1). Alternative mechanisms of new vessel development have been proposed; specifically, recruitment of blood borne progenitor cells and *in situ* vessel formation [13].

Stages of Angiogenesis

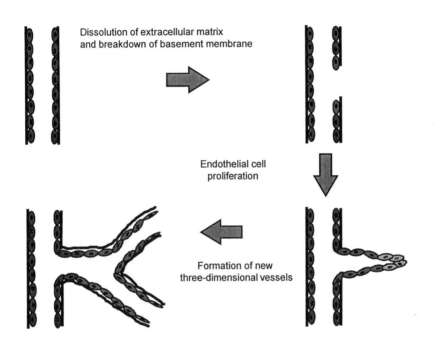

Figure 1. Stages of Angiogenesis. Cells in the local milieu stimulated by hypoxia or injury, secrete growth factors and cytokines which initiate the angiogenic process. Angiogenesis begins with the dissolution by secreted proteases of the basement membrane and extracellular matrix underlying the endothelium of the parent blood vessel, followed by endothelial cell proliferation, migration and reattachment. This culminates in the formation of three-dimensional, tube-like structures which lengthen from the tip, forming connections with other blood vessels, thus reestablishing flow.

Endothelial cells, located in capillaries, are believed to possess all the required information to form new microvascular networks [9]. Nevertheless, they do not work alone and other cell types such as mast cells, monocytes, lymphocytes, pericytes, and connective tissue cells all play a role [14-19]. Often, this role involves the expression of various growth factor proteins that in turn stimulate the replication of vital cellular components of the vasculature, such as fibroblasts, and endothelial and smooth muscle cells [14-18].

The study of angiogenesis was catalyzed by the discovery of polypeptide growth factors that are mitogenic for endothelial or other vascular-related cells *in vitro* and induce angiogenesis *in vivo*. In 1971, a tumor factor that was mitogenic for endothelial cells was first isolated [20]. This factor was subsequently determined to be one of the fibroblast growth factors [21]. Since that time, over twenty angiogenic molecules have been identified, reflecting the complex and critical nature of the angiogenic process [8].

Acidic and basic fibroblast growth factors (aFGF and bFGF) are members of a family of angiogenic proteins, which contains at least five additional polypeptides that are structurally related. aFGF (sometimes referred to as FGF-1) and bFGF (aka FGF-2) are single chain, heparin-binding polypeptides of 140 and 146 amino acids (15-17 kDa) respectively. These proteins are expressed *in vivo* by several types of cells [22]. In addition, both of the proteins have been found to be mitogenic for various cell types; for example, fibroblasts, endothelial and smooth muscle cells, myocytes and some tumor cells, all of which express at least one of the known FGF receptors [15, 21, 23, 24]. Unlike some members of the FGF family, aFGF and bFGF lack a secretory signal sequence, making the regulation of cellular secretion of these proteins unclear [24-27].

There are at least four human genes that encode for a high affinity receptor which binds aFGF and bFGF. Each of these encodes for several other receptors by alternative splicing [28, 29]. The high affinity FGF receptors possess intrinsic tyrosine kinase activity, a feature they share with other growth factor receptors. Heparan proteoglycan (located on cell surfaces) provides a low affinity binding site for aFGF and bFGF and is required for binding to their high affinity receptors [30-33].

Although vascular endothelial growth factor (VEGF - a 34-46 kDa heparin-binding, homodimeric glycoprotein [34, 35]), together with acidic and basic FGF, is expressed by many cell types, it is only a selective mitogen for endothelial cells

[36]. This singularity of expression is because of the restrictive expression by these cells of two tyrosine kinase receptors, designated *flt-1* (fms-like-tyrosine kinase) [37] and KDR/*flk-1* (kinase insert domain-containing receptor, fetal liver kinase) [38]. In addition to serving as a potent mitogen for endothelial cells, VEGF can induce permeability of capillary beds [39]. Four mRNA isoforms of VEGF (206, 189, 165 and 121 amino acid residues, respectively) are produced from a single gene by alternative splicing [36, 40, 41]. All forms of VEGF are secreted and, except for the smallest $VEGF_{121}$ isoform, all are capable of binding heparin or cell surface heparan sulfate proteoglycans [42, 43]. The heparin-binding ability of VEGF diminishes with decreasing size, such that the two larger isoforms ($VEGF_{189}$ and $VEGF_{206}$) remain membrane bound. $VEGF_{165}$ is the most abundant isoform, while $VEGF_{206}$ is the scarcest [36, 44, 45]. The $VEGF_{189}$, $VEGF_{165}$ and $VEGF_{121}$ isoforms appear to be equipotent as stimulators of angiogenesis [46].

REGULATION OF ANGIOGENESIS

Angiogenesis occurs normally during the female reproductive cycle and tissue repair following injury [14-19, 47]. Collateral vessels that "bypass" coronary obstructions have been shown to develop as a result of angiogenesis in the ischemic myocardium [12]. The angiogenesis that is thought to be induced by TMR may, in fact, be caused by myocardial injury induced by the laser [6]. Although the angiogenesis induction process that occurs during these conditions is characteristically transient and self-terminating, angiogenesis can also occur in disease states as a persistent and unregulated process. Retinal neovascularization in diabetic patients is one example of disordered angiogenesis in which capillary invasion of the vitreous humor results in subsequent hemorrhage and blindness [48]. Arthritis is characterized by synovial neovascularization and cartilage destruction, and tumor growth has been shown to be dependent on angiogenesis to supply essential substrates as increases in tumor mass result in central ischemia [49-52]. Thus, it is critical that the naturally occurring process of angiogenesis is a tightly regulated mechanism that can be stimulated by injury, ischemia or other stimulae, but is then down-regulated and/or inhibited within a time-span of days to weeks.

Although the regulation of angiogenesis is clearly complex, observations regarding the up-regulation of the growth factors and their receptors by ischemia or injury not only convey the importance of these mediators as primary stimulators of angiogenesis, but also suggest one of the basic mechanisms for regulating this process. In this regard, transient ischemia has been found to stimulate rapid up-regulation of myocardial VEGF mRNA [53, 54], and hypoxia induces up-regulation of endothelial cell expression of KDR/*flk-1* VEGF receptor [55, 56]. In a rodent model of myocardial infarction, there is up-regulation of VEGF expression as well as that of its principal receptors, KDR/*flk-1* and *flt-1* [57]. The ischemia-induced up-regulation of VEGF is regulated via a hypoxia recognition site in the promoter sequence of the VEGF gene [58].

Ischemic up-regulation of other growth factors, such as aFGF and bFGF, occurs in a fashion analogous to that for VEGF [59, 60]. The regulation of angiogenesis is, however, likely to be far more complex than that attributable simply to changes in the expression of the various growth factors and their receptors. For example, the lack of an apparent secretory mechanism for aFGF and bFGF has led to the suggestion that cell injury or death, likely events in the ischemic or traumatic conditions in which angiogenesis would be required, might cause the release of growth factors into the extracellular matrix [61]. Growth factor binding to the extracellular matrix represents another regulatory pathway. Protease up-regulation by ischemia or other stimuli, and consequent protease-mediated release of extracellular matrix-bound growth factors, which would then be readily available for stimulating angiogenesis may represent a means of activating growth factors "stored" in the extracellular matrix [62, 63]. Proteolytic enzymes may also enhance angiogenesis by allowing vascular migration into the extracellular matrix [64]. Furthermore, certain cells that express angiogenic growth factors negatively regulate angiogenesis by producing anti-angiogenic molecules, such as angiostatin [65].

Regardless of a complete understanding of the regulation of angiogenesis, one limiting aspect of this process is likely to be the limited extent and transient nature of expression of the angiogenic growth factors [54, 60, 66-68]. This observation has led to the strategy of therapeutic angiogenesis, in which exogenous angiogenic molecules are administered in order to enhance the endogenous angiogenic process. A number of growth factors have been demonstrated to enhance myocardial angiogenesis, either by administration of the protein itself or by utilizing the gene encoding for a specific angiogenic protein.

THERAPEUTIC ANGIOGENESIS

The administration of exogenous angiogenic proteins has been demonstrated to induce new blood vessel development in a number of models. In the context of the present discussion, however, only studies of therapeutic angiogenesis in the myocardium will be considered. These studies have predominantly made use of acidic FGF, basic FGF or VEGF as the angiogenic agent, although other growth factors have been utilized as well (Table 1).

Table 1. Growth factors used to induce myocardial angiogenesis

growth factor	form: route of administration	effects
aFGF	protein in collagen sponge: epicardial	smooth muscle cell hyperplasia within regions of infarction [76]
	protein in polymer: periadventitial	normalization of coronary microvascular relaxation and improved myocardial perfusion [69]
bFGF	protein: intracoronary	increased acute coronary vasodilation and increased collateralization without change in capillary density [74]. Reduction in myocardial infarct size without evidence of neovascularization [72]. Reduction in infarct size, increased perfusion and enhanced collateralization [77].
	protein in heparin-alginate beads: periadventitial	improved endothelial-dependent coronary microvascular relaxation and increased arteriolar density [71]. Reduction in infarct size and improved perfusion [75].
	protein: left atrial bolus	systemic hypotension, enhanced coronary collateralization, increased myocardial perfusion and vascular density [70,73].
FGF-5	adenoviral vector encoding FGF-5 cDNA: intracoronary	improved myocardial contractility and blood flow with histologic evidence of angiogenesis [87].
VEGF	protein: intracoronary	systemic hypotension and increased myocardial perfusion [78]. Increased myocardial perfusion and vascular density [81].
	protein: extraluminal, periadventitial	improved myocardial contractility, improved coronary blood flow and enhanced collateralization [79,80]
	protein: left atrial bolus	exacerbation of distant neointimal hyperplasia and systemic hypotension [70]

Using various experimental animal models of cardiac ischemia, a variety of administration techniques have been utilized to deliver recombinant aFGF and bFGF to the ischemic myocardium, including daily left atrial boluses, extraluminal heparin-alginate beads, calcium alginate microcapsules, intracoronary boluses, collagen type-I sponge, ethylene vinyl acetate copolymer and catheter-mediated osmotic pumps [69-77]. These studies have demonstrated enhanced collateralization to the ischemic zone, improved coronary blood flow and reduction in infarct size [69-77]. Although these results are believed to be mediated via a direct angiogenic mechanism, intracoronary delivery of bFGF in a canine temporary coronary occlusion model of infarction demonstrated a reduction in myocardial infarct size in the absence of neovascularization, suggesting myocardial salvage by unknown mechanisms that are independent of angiogenesis [72]. Further, although aFGF has been shown to be angiogenic *in vivo*, direct periadventitial application of aFGF demonstrated normalization of microvascular beta-adrenergic and endothelium-dependent relaxation, as well as increased myocardial blood flow to the ischemic region in a porcine myocardial model [69]. Furthermore, aFGF in at least one study failed to induce collateral vessel formation when applied directly to ischemic myocardial segments, but did cause vascular smooth muscle cell hyperplasia in these tissues [76].

A number of studies have also been conducted using recombinant $VEGF_{165}$ protein. In large animal models of coronary ischemia, VEGF administration, either via an intracoronary or extraluminal route, was associated with improved blood flow and function in regions of ischemia, as well as enhanced collateral vessel formation [78-81]. In contrast, systemic administration of VEGF in one study failed to result in enhanced myocardial blood flow, but did result in increased neointimal formation at a site of experimental arterial injury [70]. The mechanism underlying this outcome remains unclear, especially given the relative specificity of VEGF as an endothelial cell mitogen. One clear risk to the administration of the VEGF protein is the induction of systemic hypotension [78].

MYOCARDIAL ANGIOGENIC GENE THERAPY

Proteins such as aFGF, bFGF and VEGF are thus clearly capable of inducing angiogenesis, but the exposure of targeted tissues to these growth factors for the prolonged time periods thought to be necessary to induce therapeutic angiogenesis presents a significant challenge, especially given the requirement of sustained or repetitive delivery to an anatomically inaccessible tissue such as the ischemic myocardium. Although the use of sustained release polymers and catheter delivery systems represent potential means of sustained angiogenic protein delivery, gene therapy represents another approach that would appear ideal for circumventing the hurdle of prolonged localized protein delivery to targeted tissues. This technique, in which a cDNA encoding an angiogenic protein is delivered through one of several vectors in order to induce *in vivo* expression of the corresponding protein, has already been shown to be effective in inducing angiogenesis in experimental animal studies [46, 82-87].

Gene therapy can be defined as the introduction of exogenous genes into somatic host cells for the purposes of either replacing an absent or abnormal gene, or augmenting or over expressing a therapeutic gene product [88-90]. Over the last 10 years, more than 120 federally-approved human gene therapy trials have been directed toward the treatment of acquired and inherited disorders in a number of organ systems, including the cardiovascular system [91-93].

Approaches to somatic gene therapy can be divided into two general categories: (1) *ex vivo* gene transfer, involving the removal of cells from an organism, gene transduction *in vitro*, and reimplantation of the genetically modified cells into the appropriate tissue *in vivo*; and (2) *in vivo* gene transfer, involving the introduction of a gene into the appropriate cell type *in vivo*. The development of *ex vivo* gene transfer approaches in the heart have been limited because cardiac myocytes are terminally differentiated and have a limited life span in tissue culture, with little or no potential for cell replication [94, 95]. Recognizing these limitations, most efforts at myocardial gene transfer have focused on an *in vivo* approach.

GENE THERAPY VECTORS

A number of different methods are available for transferring DNA into cardiac myocytes: (1) plasmid DNA; (2) plasmid-liposome complexes; (3) adenovirus (Ad); (4) herpes simplex virus (HSV); and (5) adeno-associated virus (AAV). Although successful myocardial gene transfer has been accomplished with each of these methods, there are advantages and disadvantages to each.

Plasmids, genetically engineered circular double stranded DNA molecules, can be designed to contain an expression cassette for gene delivery [96]. Although plasmids were the first method described for gene transfer to myocardium [97], their level of efficiency is poor, compared with other techniques [98, 99]. By complexing the plasmid with liposomes the efficiency of gene transfer in general is improved [100]. While the liposomes used for plasmid-mediated gene transfer strategies have various compositions, they are typically synthetic cationic lipids.

The positively charged liposome forms a complex with a negatively charged plasmid. These plasmid-liposome complexes enter target cells by fusing with the plasma membrane [88, 96, 100]. Advantages of plasmid-liposome complexes include their ability to transfer large expression cassettes and their relatively low potential to evoke immunogenic responses in the host. The major disadvantage of this vector system is the low efficiency of gene transfer, requiring a large number of plasmid-liposome complexes to be presented to the target cell to obtain adequate gene transfer [96].

The adenovirus (Ad) is a 36 kb double stranded DNA virus that efficiently transfers genes *in vivo* to a variety of different target cell types, including cardiac myocytes [101]. The virus is made suitable for gene transfer by deleting the genes in the E1 region required for viral replication [102]; the expendable E3 region is also frequently deleted to allow additional room for a larger expression cassette [103]. The resulting replication deficient Ad vectors can accommodate up to 7.5 kb of exogenous genetic information [88, 103]. The vector can be produced in high titers and is capable of efficiently transferring genetic information to replicating and non-replicating cells [88,104]. This is of particular importance for transfer of genes to the myocardium, in which the host cardiac myocyte, is a terminally differentiated cell. The newly transferred genetic information remains epi-chromosomal, thus eliminating the risks of random insertional mutagenesis and permanent alteration of the genotype of the target cell [88, 101, 104]. Despite the efficiency of Ad *in vivo* gene transfer vectors, the major disadvantages of adenovirus vectors include non-specific inflammation, specific anti-Ad humoral immunity and cellular immunity to both the vector and transgene, which limit the duration of transgene expression [105-109]. Although these obstacles exist, several investigators have demonstrated that either by modifying the Ad vector or by adding immunosuppressive therapy, successful repeat administration with subsequent gene expression can be accomplished [108, 110-115].

The herpes simplex virus (HSV) is another viral vector that has been used to accomplish myocardial gene transfer [116]. The mature HSV virion consists of an enveloped icosahedral capsid with a viral genome consisting of a linear double-stranded DNA molecule that is 152 kb [117]. Most replication-deficient HSV vectors contain a deletion to remove one or more intermediate-early genes to prevent replication. Advantages of the herpes vector are its ability to enter a latent stage that could potentially result in long-term transgene expression, and its large viral DNA genome that can accommodate expression cassettes up to 25 kb [104].

Adeno-associated virus (AAV) vectors represent another potential approach to cardiovascular gene therapy. AAV is a DNA virus, which is not known to cause human disease and which requires coinfection by a helper virus (i.e. adenovirus or herpes virus) for efficient replication [118,119]. AAV vectors used for gene transfer have approximately 96% of the parental genome deleted such that only the terminal repeats remain, containing recognition signals for DNA replication and packaging [120, 121]. This allows for gene transfer while eliminating immunologic or toxic side effects due to expression of viral genes. Although prolonged myocardial expression of reporter genes has been achieved using AAV [118], several potential disadvantages to this vector system may exist, especially for angiogenic therapy, including: (1) host cell integration of the newly transferred gene and the lack of the ability to elicit a host immune response, thereby resulting in prolonged gene expression, posing the theoretical risk of excessive or inappropriate angiogenesis; (2) the difficulty in producing large titers of AAV vector relative to other vectors such as plasmid and adenovirus [122, 123].

DELIVERY STRATEGIES

A number of different strategies for the physical delivery of genetic information to myocardium have been evaluated, including: (1) direct myocardial administration; (2) indirect myocardial administration; (3) intracoronary injection through a catheter; and (4) systemic administration.

The most direct method of transferring genes to myocardium is by injection under direct vision. This can be accomplished by exposure of the myocardium through a left thoracotomy or sternotomy [124]. The advantages of a direct injection technique are the following: (1) compared with other delivery techniques, the highest levels of localized transgene expression can be achieved [98, 124, 125]; (2) vectors can be delivered with a high degree of accuracy [99,126]; (3) a number of simultaneous targeted injections can be performed [99, 126]; and (4) limited systemic spread of the vector is encountered [124]. The disadvantages of this approach are that the technique is invasive, and local inflammation at the site of vector administration has been described [97-99, 109, 127, 128].

An indirect percutaneous technique can be used in which vectors can, under radiographic control, be injected through a needle-catheter that is advanced into the left ventricular cavity and then inserted through the endocardial surface and into the myocardium [129]. Such an indirect approach, although less invasive, understandably is less precise than direct injection.

Intracoronary vector delivery involves the administration of vectors through coronary catheters that are placed percutaneously. The principal advantages of this technique are that it is relatively non-invasive and is believed to induce less of a localized inflammatory response than a direct injection [87, 124, 130, 131]. The disadvantages of this strategy are that lower levels of transgene expression are achieved compared with direct injection [124, 125], and some degree of systemic spread of the vector is encountered [87, 130].

Myocardial gene transfer following systemic delivery of vectors has also been described. Intravenous [132] administrations of Ad vectors have resulted in measurable myocardial transgene expression, albeit far less than by direct administration [124]. The obvious disadvantage of this technique is that, by definition, profound systemic spread occurs. The utilization of myocardial-specific promoters, however, such as the myosin heavy chain promoter [126, 133-136], could potentially permit more site-specific gene transfer following a systemic delivery.

EFFICACY OF MYOCARDIAL ANGIOGENIC GENE THERAPY

Several studies have now been published regarding the efficacy of delivery to the heart of a cDNA encoding for an angiogenic protein. In one study, direct injection of a plasmid expressing FGF-5 into rodent myocardium resulted in increased capillary density compared with controls [137]. In a canine model, a single direct myocardial injection of an Ad vector expressing VEGF resulted in sustained levels of localized VEGF protein for at least seven days after vector administration [124]. Importantly, VEGF expression was localized to the myocardium, and the direct myocardial injections did not effect global or regional ventricular function in this study. In a porcine model of myocardial ischemia, a single intracoronary administration of an Ad vector expressing FGF-5 resulted in detectable levels of FGF-5 mRNA in the myocardium fourteen days after vector administration, and contrast echocardiography demonstrated increased wall thickening and improved blood flow in the ischemic zone two and twelve weeks after vector administration [87]. Finally, we have recently demonstrated significantly improved perfusion and contractile function in ischemic porcine myocardium utilizing an adenovirus vector encoding the cDNA for human $VEGF_{121}$ [138].

CONCLUSIONS

Angiogenesis is a complex biological process, mediated by a number of identified angiogenic proteins, occurs in a variety of normal and pathological conditions, and may be an important component underlying the efficacy of TMR. Therapeutic angiogenesis describes a clinical strategy of administering an angiogenic growth factor in order to enhance the endogenous angiogenic processes. Gene therapy is a novel delivery strategy that may be useful in inducing therapeutic angiogenesis, especially in such inaccessible tissues as the myocardium. If angiogenesis does prove to be a critical component of TMR, therapeutic angiogenesis, induced either by protein or gene delivery, may ultimately become an important adjunct to this technique. Each of these strategies may serve as an important alternative or adjunctive therapy in individuals with coronary artery disease.

References

1. Kannel WB. Incidence, prevalence and mortality of coronary artery disease. In Fuster V, Ross R and Topol E (eds). Atherosclerosis and Coronary Artery Disease. Philadelphia, Lippincott; 1996, pp. 13-24.
2. Centers for Disease Control and Prevention: National Center for Health Statistics, National Vital Statistics and The United States Bureau of the Census. Health, United States 1993, p. 31.
3. Mirhoseini M, Cayton M. Revascularization of the heart by laser. J Microsurg 1981;2:253-260.
4. Okada M, Shimizu K, Ikuta H, Horii H, Nakamura K. A new method of myocardial revascularization by laser. J Thorac Cardiovasc Surg 1992;39:1-4.
5. Cooley DA, Frazier OH, Kadipasaoglu KA, Pehlivanoglu S, Shannon RL, Angelini P. Transmyocardial laser revascularization: anatomic evidence of long-term channel patency. Texas Heart Inst J 1994;21:220-224.
6. Zlotnick AY, Ahmad RM, Reul RM, Laurence RG, Aretz HT, Cohn LH. Neovascularization occurs at the site of closed laser channels after transmyocardial laser revascularization. Surg Forum 1996;47:286-287.
7. Mack CA, Magovern CJ, Hahn RT, Sanborn T, Ko W, Isom OW, Rosengart TK. Channel patency and neovascularization following transmyocardial revascularization utilizing an excimer laser: results and comparisons to non-lased channels. Circulation 1996;94 (Suppl. 1):I-294. (abstract)
8. Folkman J, Klagsbrun M. A Family of Angiogenic Peptides. Nature 1987;329: 671-672.
9. Folkman J, Haudenschild C. Angiogenesis *in vitro*. Nature 1980;288:551-556.
10. Dumont DJ, Fong G-H, Puri MC, Gradwohl G, Alitalo D, Breitman ML. Vascularization of the mouse embryo: a study of flk-1, tek, tie and vascular endothelial growth factor expression during development. Dev Dyn 1995;203:80-92.
11. Gilbert SF. Developmental Biology, 3rd ed. Sunderland, MA. Sinauer Associates, 1991:891.
12. Schaper W, Ito W. Molecular Mechanisms of Coronary Collateral Vessel Growth. Circ Res 1996;79:911-919.
13. Asahara T, Murohara T, Sullivan A, Silver M, van der Zee R, Li T, Witzenbichler B, Schatteman G, Isner J. Isolation of putative progenitor endothelial cells for angiogenesis. Science 1997;275:964-967.
14. Folkman J. Angiogenesis in cancer, vascular, rheumatoid and other diseases. Nature Med 1995;1:27-31.
15. Folkman J, Shing Y. Angiogenesis. J Biol Chem 1992;267:10931-10934.
16. Klagsbrun M, Folkman J. Angiogenesis. In: Sporn MB, Roberts AB (eds) Peptide growth factors and their receptors II. 1990. Springer, Berlin, Heidelberg, New York, pp549-574.
17. Montesano R. 1992 Mack Forster Award Lecture. Review. Regulation of angiogenesis *in vitro*. Eur J Clin Invest 1992;22:504-515.

18. Risau W. Angiogenic growth factors. Prog Growth Factor Res 1990;2:71-79 .
19. Weinstat-Saslow D, Steeg PS. Angiogenesis and colonization in the tumor metastatic process: basic and applied advances. FASEB J 1994;8:401-407.
20. Folkman J, Merler E, Abernathy C, Williams G. Isolation of a tumor factor responsible for angiogenesis. J Exp Med 1971;133:275-288.
21. Gospodarowicz D, Ferrara N, Schweigerer L, Neufeld G. Structural characterization and biologic functions of fibroblast growth factor. Endocrine Rev 1987;8:95-114.
22. Burgess WH, Maciag T. The heparin-binding (fibroblast) growth factor family of proteins. Ann Rev Biochem 1989;58:575-606 .
23. Brindle NPJ. Growth factors in endothelial regeneration. Cardiovasc Res 1993;27:1162-1172.
24. Baird A, Bohlen P. Fibroblast Growth Factors. In; Sporn MB, Roberts AD (eds) Peptide Growth Factors and Their Receptors I. 1990 Springer, Berlin Heidelberg New York, pp369-418.
25. Kandel J, Bossy-Wentzel E, Radvanyi F, Klagsbrun M, Folkman J, Hanahan D. Neovascularization is associated with a switch to the export of bFGF in the multistep development of fibrosarcoma. Cell 1991;66:1095-1104.
26. Jaye M, Howk R, Burgess W, Ricca GA, Chiu IM, Ravera MW, O'Brien SJ, Modi WS, Maciag T, Drohan WN. Human endothelial cell growth factor: cloning, nucleotide sequence, and chromosome location. Science 1986;233:541-545 .
27. Abraham JA, Mergia A, Whang JL, Tumolo A, Friedman J, Hjerrild KA, Gospodarowicz D, Fiddes JC. Nucleotide sequence of a bovine clone encoding the angiogenic protein, basic fibroblast growth factor. Science 1986;233:545-548.
28. Houssaint E, Blanquet P, Champion-Arnoud P, Gesnel MC, Torriglia A, Courtois Y, Breathnach R. Related fibroblast growth factor receptor genes exist in the human genome. Proc Natl Acad Sci USA 1990;87:8180-8184.
29. Johnson D, Lee P, Lu J, Williams L. Diverse forms of a receptor for acidic and basic fibroblast growth factors. Mol Cell Biol 1990;10:4728-4736.
30. Moscatelli D. Metabolism of receptor-bound and matrix-bound basic fibroblast growth by bovine capillary endothelial cells. J Cell Biol 1988;107:753-759.
31. Yayon A, Klagsbrun M, Esko J, Leder P, Ornitz D. Cell surface heparin-like molecules are required for binding of basic fibroblast growth factor to its high affinity receptor. Cell 1991;64:841-848.
32. Brown KJ, Hendry IA, Parish CR. Acidic and basic fibroblast growth factor bind with differing affinity to the same heparan sulfate proteoglycan on BALB/c 3T3 cells: implications for potentiation of growth factor action by heparin. J Cell Biochem 1995;58:6-14.
33. Reich-Slotky R, Bonneh-Barkay D, Shaoul E, Bluma B, Svahn CM, Ron D. Differential effect of cell-associated heparan sulfates on the binding of keratinocyte growth factor (KGF) and acidic fibroblast growth factor to the KGF receptor. J Biol Chem 1994;269:32279-32285.
34. Gospodarowicz D, Abraham J, Schilling J. Isolation and characterization of a vascular endothelial cell mitogen produced by pituitary-derived folliculo stellate

cells. Proc Natl Acad Sci USA 1989;86:7311-7315.

35. Ferrara N, Henzel WJ. Pituitary follicular cells secrete a novel heparin-binding growth factor specific for vascular endothelial cells. Biochem Biophys Res Commun 1989;161:851-858.

36. Ferrara N, Houck K, Jakeman L, Winer J, Leung D. The vascular endothelial growth factor family of polypeptides. J Cell Biochem 1991;47:211-218.

37. Shibuya M, Yamaguchi S, Yamane A, Ikeda T, Tojo A, Matsushime H, Sato M. Nucleotide sequence and expression of a novel human receptor-type tyrosine kinase gene (flt) closely related to the fms family. Oncogene 1990;5:519-524.

38. Terman B, Dougher-Vermazen M, Carrion M, Dimitrov D, Armellino D, Gospodarowicz D, Bohlen P. Identification of the KDR tyrosine kinase as a receptor for vascular endothelial growth factor. Biochem Biophys Res Commun 1992;187:1579-1586.

39. Neufeld G, Tessler S, Gitay-Goren H, Cohen T, Levi B-Z. Vascular endothelial growth factor and its receptors. Prog Growth Factor Res 1994;5:89-97.

40. Leung D, Cachianes G, Kuang W-J, Goeddel D, Ferrara N. Vascular endothelial growth factor is a secreted angiogenic mitogen. Science 1989;246:1306-1309.

41. Tischer E, Gospodarowicz D, Mitchell R, Silva M, Schilling J, Lau K, Crisp T, Fiddes JC, Abraham JA. Vascular endothelial growth factor: a new member of the platelet-derived growth factor gene family. Biochem Biophys Res Commun 1989;165:1198-1206.

42. Houck KA, Ferrara N, Winer J, Cachianes G, Li B, Leung DW. The vascular endothelial growth factor family: identification of a fourth molecular species and characterization of alternative splicing of RNA. Mol Endocrinol 1991;5:1806-1814.

43. Houck KA, Leung DW, Rowland AM, Winer J, Ferrara N. Dual regulation of vascular endothelial growth factor bioavailability by genetic and proteolytic mechanisms. J Biol Chem 1992;267:26031-26037 .

44. Tischer E, Mitchell R, Hartman T, Silva M, Gospodarowicz D, Fiddes J, Abraham J. The Human gene for vascular endothelial growth factor. Multiple protein forms are encoded through alternative exon splicing. J Biol Chem 1991;266:11947-11954.

45. Park J, Keller G-A, Ferrara N. The vascular endothelial growth factor (VEGF) isoforms: differential deposition into the subepithelial extracellular matrix and bioactivity of extracellular matrix-bound VEGF. Mol Biol Chem 1993;4:1317-1326.

46. Takeshita S, Yukio T, Thierry C, Takayuki A, Bauters C, Symes J, Ferrara N, Isner J. Gene transfer of naked DNA encoding for three isoforms of vascular endothelial growth factor stimulates collateral development *in vivo*. Lab Invest 1996;75:487-501.

47. Liotta LA, Steeg PS, Stetler-Stevenson WG. Cancer metastasis and angiogenesis: an imbalance of positive and negative regulation. Cell 1991;64:327-336.

48. Folkman J. 11th Congress of Thrombosis and Haemostasis (Verstraete M, Vermylen J, Lignen R, Arnout J, eds) pp583-596, Leuven University Press, Leuven.

49. Peacock DJ, Banquerigo ML, Brahn E. Angiogenesis inhibition suppresses

collagen arthritis. J Exp Med 1992;175:1135-1138.

50. Folkman J, Watson K, Ingber D, Hanahan D. Induction of angiogenesis during the transition from hyperplasia to neoplasia. Nature 1989;339:58-61.
51. Weidner N, Semple J, Welch W, Folkman J. Tumor angiogenesis correlates with metastasis in invasive breast carcinoma. N Engl J Med 1991;324:1-8.
52. Folkman J. Angiogenesis and breast cancer. J Clin Oncol 1994;12:441-443.
53. Sharma HS, Sassen L, Knoll R, Verdouw PD. Myocardial expression of vascular endothelial growth factor: enhanced transcription during ischemia and reperfusion. Circulation 1992;86 (suppl I):I-1168. (abstract)
54. Banai S, Shweiki D, Pinson A, Chandra M, Lazarovici G, Keshet E. Upregulation of vascular endothelial growth factor expression induced by myocardial ischaemia: implications for coronary angiogenesis. Cardiovasc Res 1994;28:1176-1179.
55. Waltenberger J, Mayr U, Pentz S, Hombach V. Functional upregulation of the vascular endothelial growth factor receptor KDR by hypoxia. Circulation 1996;94:1647-1654.
56. Brogi E, Schatteman G, Wu T, Kim E, Varticovski L, Keyt B, Isner J. Hypoxia-induced paracrine regulation of vascular endothelial growth factor receptor expression. J Clin Invest. 1996;97:469-476.
57. Li J, Brown L, Hibberd M, Grossman J, Morgan J, Simons M. VEGF, *flk-1*, and *flt-1* expression in a rat myocardial infarction model of angiogenesis. Am J Physiol 1996;270:H1803-H1811.
58. Ikeda E, Achen MG, Breier G, Risau W. Hypoxia-induced transcriptional activation and increased mRNA stability of vascular endothelial growth factor in C6 glioma cells. J Biol Chem 1995;270:19761-19766.
59. Kuwabara K, Ogawa S, Matsumoto M, Koga S, Clauss M, Pinsky DJ, Lyn P, Leavy J, Witte L, Joseph-Silverstein J, et al. Hypoxia-mediated induction of acidic/basic fibroblast growth factor and platelet-derived growth factor in mononuclear phagocytes stimulates growth of hypoxic endothelial cells. Proc Natl Acad Sci USA 1995;92:4606-4610.
60. Rosengart T, Duenas M, Winkles J, Krieger K, Isom OW. Ischemia is associated with increased expression of the angiogenic protein acidic fibroblast growth factor: implications for "biologic" revascularization. Surg Forum 1994;45:392-395.
61. Gajdusek CM, Carbon S. Injury induced release of basic fibroblast growth factor from bovine aortic endothelial cells. J Cell Physiol 1989;139:570-579.
62. Saksela O, Rifkin DB. Release of basic fibroblast growth factor-heparan sulfate complexes from endothelial cells by plasminogen activator-mediated proteolytic activity. J Cell Biol 1990;110:767-775.
63. Ishai-Michaeli R, Eldor A, Vlodavsky I. Heparanase activity expressed by platelets, neutrophils and lymphoma cells releases active fibroblast growth factor from extracellular matrix. Cell Regul 1990;1:833-842 .
64. Klagsbrun M, D'Amore PA. Regulators of angiogenesis. Ann Rev Physiol 1991; 53:217-239.
65. O'Reilly MA, Holmgren L, Shing Y, Chen C, Rosenthal RA, Moses M, Lane WS, Cao Y, Sage EH, Folkman J. Angiostatin: a novel angiogenesis inhibitor that

mediates the suppression of metastases by a Lewis lung carcinoma. Cell 1994; 79:315-328.

66. Shweiki D, Itin A, Soffer D, Keshet E. Vascular endothelial growth factor induced by hypoxia may mediate hypoxia-initiated angiogenesis. Nature 1992;359:843-845.

67. Hashimoto E, Ogita T, Nakaoka T, Matsuoka R, Takao A, Kira Y. Rapid induction of vascular endothelial growth factor expression by transient ischemia in rat heart. Am J Physiol 1994;267:H1948-H1954.

68. Brogi E, Wu T, Namiki A, Isner JM. Indirect angiogenic cytokines upregulate VEGF and bFGF gene expression in vascular smooth muscle cells, whereas hypoxia upregulates VEGF expression only. Circulation 1994;90:649-652.

69. Sellke F, Li J, Stamler A, Lopez J, Thomas K, Simons M. Angiogenesis induced by acidic fibroblast growth factor as an alternative method of revascularization for chronic myocardial ischemia. Surgery 1996;120:182-188.

70. Lazarous DF, Shou M, Scheinowitz H, Hodge E, Thirumurti V, Kitsiou AN, Stiber JA, Lobo AD, Hunsberger S, Guetta E, Epstein SE, Unger EF. Comparative effects of basic fibroblast growth factor and vascular endothelial growth factor on coronary collateral development and the arterial response to injury. Circulation 1996; 94: 1074-1082.

71. Sellke FW, Wang SY, Friedman M, Harada K, Edelman ER, Grossman W, Simons M. Basic FGF enhances endothelium-dependent relaxation of the collateral-perfused coronary microcirculation. Am J Physiol 1994;267:H1303-H1311.

72. Horrigan M, MacIsaac A, Nicolini F, Vince D, Lee P, Ellis S, Topol E. Reduction in myocardial infarct size by basic fibroblast growth factor after temporary coronary occlusion in a canine model. Circulation 1996;94:1927-1933.

73. Lazarous DF, Scheinowitz M, Shou M, Hodge E, Rajanayagam S, Hunsberger S, Robison WG Jr., Stiber JA, Correa R, Epstein SE, et al. Effects of chronic systemic administration of basic fibroblast growth factor on collateral development in the canine heart. Circulation 1995;91:145-153.

74. Unger E, Banai S, Shou M, Lazarous D, Jaklitsch M, Scheinowitz M, Correa R, Klingbeil C, Epstein S. Basic fibroblast growth factor enhances myocardial collateral flow in a canine model. Am J Physiol 1994;266:H1588-H1595.

75. Harada K, Grossman W, Friedman M, Edelman E, Prasad P, Keighley C, Manning W, Sellke F, Simons M. Basic fibroblast growth factor improves myocardial function in chronically ischemic porcine hearts. J Clin Invest 1994;94:623-630.

76. Banai S, Jaklitsch MT, Casscells W, Shou M, Shrivastav S, Correa R, Epstein SE, Unger EF. Effects of acidic fibroblast growth factor on normal and ischemic myocardium. Circ Res 1991;69:76-85.

77. Yanagisawa-Miwa A, Uchida Y, Nakamura F, Tomaru T, Kido H, Kamijo T, Sugimoto T, Kaji K, Utsuyama M, Kurashima C, et al. Salvage of infarcted myocardium by angiogenic action of basic fibroblast growth factor. Science 1992;257:1401-1403.

78. Hariawala M, Horowitz J, Esakof D, Sherrif D, Walter D, Keyt B, Isner J, Symes J. VEGF improves myocardial blood flow but produces EDRF-mediated hypotension in porcine hearts. J Surg Res 1996;63:77-82 .

79. Harada K, Friedman M, Lopez JJ, Wang SY, Li J, Prasad PV, Pearlman JD, Edelman ER, Selke FW, Simons M. Vascular endothelial growth factor administration in chronic myocardial ischemia. Am J Physiol 1996;270:H1791-H1802.

80. Pearlman JD, Hibberd MG, Chuang ML, Harada K, Lopez JJ, Gladstone SR, Friedman M, Sellke FW, Simons M. Magnetic resonance mapping demonstrates benefits of VEGF-induced myocardial angiogenesis. Nature Med 1995;1: 1085-1089.

81. Banai S, Jaklitsch MT, Shou M, Lazarous DF, Scheinowitz M, Biro S, Epstein SE, Unger EF. Angiogenic-induced enhancement of collateral blood flow to ischemic myocardium by vascular endothelial growth factor in dogs. Circulation 1994;89: 2183-2189.

82. Magovern CJ, Mack CA, Zhang J, Rosengart TK, Isom OW, Crystal RG. Regional angiogenesis induced in non-ischemic tissue by an adenoviral vector expressing vascular endothelial growth factor. Hum Gene Ther 1997;8:215-227.

83. Muhlhauser J, Pili R, Merril MJ, Maeda H, Passaniti A, Crystal RG, Capogrossi MC. In vivo angiogenesis induced by recombinant adenovirus vectors coding either for secreted or non-secreted forms of acidic fibroblast growth factor. Hum Gene Ther 1995;6:1457-1465.

84. Mühlhauser J, Merrill MJ, Pili R, Maeda H, Bacic M, Bewig B, Passaniti A, Edwards NA, Crystal RG, Capogrossi MC. VEGF$_{165}$ expressed by a replication-deficient recombinant adenovirus vector induces angiogenesis in vivo. Circ Res 1995;77: 1077-1086.

85. Mesri EA, Federoff HJ, Brownlee M. Expression of vascular endothelial growth factor from a defective herpes simplex virus type 1 amplicon vector induces angiogenesis in mice. Circ Res 1995;76:161-167.

86. Tsurumi Y, Takeshita S, Chen D, Kearney M, Rossow ST, Passeri J, Horowitz JR, Symes JF, Isner JF. Direct intramuscular gene transfer of naked DNA encoding vascular endothelial growth factor augments collateral development and tissue perfusion. Circulation 1996;94:3281-3290.

87. Giordano FJ, Ping P, Mckirnan MD, Nozaki S, DeMaria AN, Dillmann WH, Mathieu-Costello O, Hammond HK. Intracoronary gene transfer of fibroblast growth factor-5 increases blood flow and contractile function in an ischemic region of the heart. Nature Med 1996;2:534-539.

88. Miller AD. Human gene therapy comes of age. Nature 1992;357:455-60.

89. Anderson WF. Human gene therapy. Science 1992;256:808-13.

90. Mulligan RC. The basic science of gene therapy. Science 1993;260:926-32.

91. Human gene marker/therapy clinical protocols. Hum Gene Ther 1996;7:567-586.

92. Isner JM. Arterial gene transfer for therapeutic angiogenesis in patients with peripheral artery disease. Human Gene Ther 1996;7:959-88.

93. Isner JM, Pieczek A, Schainfeld R, Blair R, Haley L, Asahara T, Rosenfield K, Razvi S, Walsh K, Symes JF. Clinical evidence of angiogenesis after arterial gene transfer of phVEGF165 in patient with ischaemic limb. Lancet. 1996;348:370-374.

94. Zack R. Development and proliferation capacity of cardiac muscle cells. Circ Res

1974; 34-35 (suppl II):II-17.

95. Wantanabe AM, Green FJ, Farmer BB. Preparation and use of cardiac myocytes in experimental cardiology. In: The Heart and Cardiovascular System. Fozzard HA, Haber E, Jennings RB, Katz AM, Morgan HE, eds. New York: 1988; Raven Press.

96. Crystal RG. Transfer of genes to humans: Early lessons and obstacles to success. Science 1995;270: 404-410.

97. Lin H, Parmacek MS, Morle G, Bolling S, Leiden JM. Expression of recombinant genes in myocardium *in vivo* after direct injection of DNA. Circulation 1990;82: 2217-2221.

98. Guzman RJ, Lemarchand P, Crystal RG, Epstein SE, Finkel T. Efficient gene transfer into myocardium by direct injection of adenovirus vectors. Circ Res 1993;73:12202-1207.

99. French BA, Mazur W, Geske RS, Bolli R. Direct *in vivo* gene transfer into porcine myocardium using replication-deficient adenoviral vectors. Circulation 1994;90 :2414-2424.

100. Nicolau C, LePape A, Soriano P, Fargette F, Juhel MF. *In vivo* expression of rat insulin after intravenous administration of the liposome-entrapped gene for rat insulin I. Proc Natl Acad Sci USA 1983;80:1068-72.

101. Horwitz MS. Adenoviruses. In: Fields Virology. Fields BN, Knipe DM, Howley PM, eds. Philadelphia: 1996, Lippincott-Raven Publishers, pp 2149-71.

102. Graham FL, Smiley J, Russell WC, Nairn R. Characteristics of a human cell line transformed by DNA from human adenovirus type 5. J Gen Virol 1977;36:59-74.

103. Graham FL. Manipulation of adenovirus vectors. In: Methods in Molecular Biology. Murray EJ (ed). Clifton: 1991, The Humana Press, pp 109-28.

104. Ali M, Lemoine NR, Ring CJ. The use of DNA viruses as vectors for gene therapy. Gene Ther 1994;1:367-84.

105. Yang Y, Nunes FA, Berencsi K, Furth EE, Gonczol E, Wilson JM. Cellular immunity to viral antigens limits E1-deleted adenoviruses for gene therapy. Proc Natl Acad Sci 1994;91:4407-4411.

106. Yang Y, Li Q, Ertl HCJ, Wilson JM. Cellular and humoral immune responses to viral antigens create barriers to lung-directed gene therapy with recombinant adenoviruses. J Virol 1995;69:2004-2015.

107. Yang Y, Joos KU, Su Q, Ertl HCJ, Wilson JM. Immune responses to viral antigens versus transgene product in the elimination of recombinant adenovirus-infected hepatocytes *in vivo*. Gene Ther 1996;3:137-144.

108. Mack CA, Song WR, Carpenter HC, Wickham T, Kovesdi I, Harvey BG, Magovern CJ, Isom OW, Rosengart TK, Falck-Pedersen E, Hackett NR, Crystal RG, Mastrangeli A. Circumvention of anti-adenovirus neutralizing immunity by administration of an adenoviral vector of an alternate serotype. Human Gene Ther 1997;8:99-109.

109. Quinones MJ, Leor J, Kloner RA, Ito M, Patterson M, Witke WF, Kedes L. Avoidance of immune response prolongs expression of genes delivered to the adult rat myocardium by replication-defective adenovirus. Circulation 1996;94:1394-1401.

110. Kass-Eisler A, Leinwand L, Gall J, Bloom B, Falck-Pedersen E. Circumventing the immune response to adenovirus-mediated gene therapy. Gene Ther 1996;3:154-162.
111. Mastrangeli A, Harvey BG, Yao J, Wolf G, Kovesdi I, Crystal RG, Falck-Pedersen E. "Sero-switch" adenovirus-mediated *in vivo* gene transfer: circumvention of anti-adenovirus humoral immune defenses against repeat administration by changing the adenovirus serotype. Human Gene Ther 1996;7:79-87.
112. Gilgenkrantz H, Duboc D, Juillard V, Couton D, Pavirani A, Guillet JG, Briand P, Khan A. Transient expression of genes transferred *in vivo* into heart using first-generation adenoviral vectors: role of the immune response. Human Gene Ther 1995;6:1265-1274.
113. Kay MA, Holterman AX, Meuse L, Gown A, Och HD, Linsley PS, Wilson CB. Long-term hepatic adenovirus-mediated gene expression in mice following CTLA4lg administration. Nature Genet 1995;11:191-197.
114. Yang Y, Nunes FA, Berencsi K, Gonczol E, Engelhardt JF, Wilson JM. Inactivation of E2a in recombinant adenoviruses improves the prospect for gene therapy in cystic fibrosis. Nature Genet 1994;7:362-369.
115. Yang Y, Greenough K, Wilson JM. Transient immune blockade prevents formation of neutralizing antibody to recombinant adenovirus and allows repeated gene transfer to mouse liver. Gene Ther 1996;3:412-420.
116. Coffin RS, Howard MK, Cumming DVE, Dollery CM, McEwan J, Yellon DM, Marber MS, MacLean AR, Brown SM, Latchman DS. Gene delivery to the heart *in vivo* and to cardiac myocytes and smooth muscle cells *in vitro* using herpes virus vectors. Gene Ther 1996;3:560-566.
117. Glorioso JC, DeLuca NA, Fink DJ. Development and application of herpes simplex virus vectors for human gene therapy. Annu Rev Microbiol 1995;49: 675-710.
118. Kaplitt MG, Xiao X, Samulski RJ, Li J, Ojamaa K, Klein IL, Makimura H, Kaplitt MJ, Strumpf RK, Diethrich EB. Long-term gene transfer in porcine myocardium after coronary infusion of an adeno-associated virus vector. Ann Thorac Surg 1996;62:1669-1676.
119. Lebkowski JS, McNally MM, Okarma TB, Lerch LB. Adeno-associated virus: a vector system for efficient introduction and integration of DNA into a variety of mammalian cell types. Mol Cell Biol 1988;8:3988-3996.
120. SamulskI RJ, Chang LS, Shenk T. A recombinant plasmid from which an infectious adeno-associated virus genome can be excised *in vitro* and its use to study viral replication. J Virol 1987;61:3096-3101.
121. SamulskI RJ, Chang LS, Shenk T. Helper-free stocks of adeno-associated viruses: normal integration does not require viral gene expression. J Virol 1989;63:3822-3828.
122. Kotin RM. Prospects for the use of adeno-associated virus as a vector for human gene therapy. Human Gene Ther 1994;5:793-801.
123. Flotte TR, Carter BJ. Adeno-associated virus vectors for gene therapy. Gene Ther 1995;2:357-362.
124. Magovern CJ, Mack CA, Zhang J, Hahn RT, Ko W, Isom OW, Crystal RG, Rosengart TK. Direct *in vivo* gene transfer to canine myocardium using a

replication-deficient adenovirus vector. Ann Thorac Surg 1996;62:425-434.

125. Muhlhauser J, Jones M, Yamada I, Cirielli C, Lemarchand P, Gloe TR, Bewig B, Signoretti S, Crystal RG, Capogrossi MC. Safety and efficacy of *in vivo* gene transfer into the porcine heart with replication-deficient, recombinant adenovirus vectors. Gene Therapy 1996;3:145-153.

126. von Harsdorf R, Schott RJ, Shen YT, Vatner SF, Mahdavi V, Nadal-Ginard B. Gene injection into canine myocardium as a useful model for studying gene expression in the heart of large mammals. Circ Res 1993;72:688-695.

127. Gal D, Weir L, Leclerc G, Pickering JG, Hogan J, Isner JM. Direct myocardial transfection in two animal models. Evaluation of parameters affecting gene expression and percutaneous gene delivery. Lab Invest 1993;68:18-25.

128. Kass-Eisler A, Falck-Pedersen E, Alvira M, Rivera J, Buttrick PM, Wittenberg BA, Cipriani L, Leinwand LA. Quantitative determination of adenovirus-mediated gene delivery to rat cardiac myocytes *in vitro* and *in vivo*. Proc Natl Acad Sci USA 1993;90:11498-11502.

129. Li JJ, Ueno H, Pan Y, Tomita H, Yamamoto H, Kanegae Y, Saito I, Takeshita A. Percutaneous transluminal gene transfer into canine myocardium *in vivo* by replication-defective adenovirus. Cardiovasc Res 1995;30:97-105.

130. Barr E, Carroll J, Kalynych AM, Tripathy SK, Kozarsky K, Wilson JM. Efficient catheter-mediated gene transfer into the heart using replication- defective adenovirus. Gene Ther 1994;1:51-58.

131. Gojo S, Niwaya K, Yoshida Y, Kawachi K, Kitamura S. *Ex vivo* adenovirus mediated gene transfer into transplanted hearts. J Heart Lung Trans 1996;15:S63.

132. Stratford-Perricaudet LD, Makeh I, Perricaudet M, Briand P. Widespread long-term gene transfer to mouse skeletal muscles and heart. J Clin Invest 1992;90:626-630.

133. Kitsis RN, Buttrick PM, McNally EM, Kaplan ML, Leinwand LA. Hormonal modulation of a gene injected into rat heart *in vivo*. Proc Natl Acad Sci USA 1991;88:4138-4142.

134. Buttrick PM, Kass A, Kitsis RN, Kaplan ML, Leinwand LA. Behavior of genes directly injected into the rat heart *in vivo*. Circ Res 1992;70:193-198.

135. Fishman GI, Kaplan ML, Buttrick PM. Tetracycline-regulated cardiac gene expression *in vivo*. J Clin Invest 1994;93:1864-1868.

136. Prentice H, Kloner RA, Prigozy T, Christensen T, Newman L, Li Y, Kedes L. Tissue restricted gene expression assayed by direct DNA injection into cardiac and skeletal muscle. J Mol Cell Cardiol 1994;26:1393-1401.

137. Barr E, Lin H, Bolling S, Engelmann GL, Leiden JM. Induction of angiogenesis following *in vivo* gene transfer into the myocardium. Circulation 1991;84 Supplement:II-420

138. Mack CA, Patel SR, Schwarz EA, Zanzonico P, Hahn RT, Ilercil A, Devereux RB, Goldsmith SJ, Christian TF, Sanborn TA, Kovesdi I, Isom OW, Crystal RG, Rosengart TK. Myocardial perfusion and function following adenovirus-mediated transfer of the $VEGF_{121}$ cDNA to the ischemic porcine myocardium. Abstract. American Association for Thoracic Surgery, 1997.

Index